Primary Care Diagnostics
Second Edition

Primary Care Diagnostics

The patient-centred approach in the new commissioning environment

Second Edition

Nicholas Summerton

General Practitioner, Yorkshire

Radcliffe Publishing
London • New York

HEAL

Radcliffe Publishing Ltd
33-41 Dallington Street
London EC1V 0BB
Tel: 020 7954 3400
Fax: 020 7253 5946

www.radcliffepublishing.com

Electronic catalogue and worldwide online ordering facility.

British Library Cataloguing in Publication Data

A catalogue record for this book is available from the British Library.

ISBN-10: 1846195047
ISBN-13: 9781846195044

Typeset by KnowledgeWorks Global Ltd, Chennai, India
Printed and bound by Cadmus Communications, USA

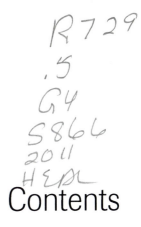

Contents

Preface to the second edition

This book was originally published back in 2007 with the title *'Patient Centred Diagnosis'*. However, in writing a revised second edition and including two new chapters on cancer and commissioning, it became clear that *'Primary Care Diagnostics'* would be a more appropriate title. This means not that the patient-centred element has been downgraded in any way, but rather that there are a number of equally important issues that need to be considered by clinicians or commissioners focusing on the diagnostic approach within primary care. These are:

- maintaining a broad and patient-centred approach
- being alert to the importance of context and its impact on the validity and the reliability of all clinical information
- using information obtained from the medical history and the clinical examination wisely
- harnessing the diagnostic processing pathway both for clinical care and for commissioning
- focusing on patient-oriented and health service outcomes
- appreciating the unique nature of primary care decision making in relation to, for example, precision and uncertainty
- adopting distinct diagnostic strategies such as the 'test of time'
- ensuring the appropriate and efficient use of investigations combined with clarity about the purpose of any test

This book is written from the perspective of a practising general practitioner who also has a clinical research interest in diagnostics. In the academic tradition, I have assimilated and discussed a wealth of evidence but, as a primary care clinician, I have also sought to place such information in context. The book is also deliberately personalised: scattered throughout the text are real examples of my own mistakes, concerns and dilemmas (together with the rarer success!).

Nick Summerton
December 2010

Preface to the first edition

In recent years academic primary care has become increasingly colonised by those who don't see patients or can't see patients. Although such individuals obviously make few clinical errors compared to the rest of us, the broader consequences are potentially disastrous. Primary care clinical research and development is being side-lined and researchers often seem more concerned about publications than patients. Even more worryingly, in some key clinical areas such as diagnostics, politicians and policy makers seem to have adopted the views and values of such non-clinical academics.

This book is written from the perspective of a practising general practitioner who also has a clinical research interest in diagnostics. In the academic tradition, I have assimilated and discussed a wealth of evidence but, as a primary care clinician, I have also sought to place such information in context. The book is deliberately personalised: scattered throughout the text are real examples of my mistakes, concerns and dilemmas (together with the rarer successes!). By the end of the book I hope the reader will be able to picture me sitting in my surgery in Yorkshire seeing a patient, rather than in an empty office with a computer!

Nick Summerton
September 2006

About the author

Dr Nick Summerton is a general practitioner and a public health physician. Following five years working in single-handed practice in Huddersfield he underwent further training in epidemiology in the UK and in Canada. Subsequently he has worked in East Yorkshire as a part-time general practitioner and also as a senior lecturer/reader in primary care medicine. During this time he has developed a specific research interest in primary care diagnostics, gaining a doctorate from the University of Oxford in 2003.

Dr Summerton has an extensive publication record in both research and educational journals. His other books are *Diagnosing Cancer in Primary Care* (1999) and *Medicine and Health Care in Roman Britain* (2007). He is a member of the Department of Health's National Imaging Board and the Diagnostic Advisory Committee at the National Institute for Health and Clinical Excellence (NICE).

Acknowledgements

In developing the ideas contained in this book I am particularly grateful to Professor David Mant (University of Oxford), Professor Peter Campion (University of Hull), Professor J André Knottnerus (University of Maastricht) and Professor Ian McWhinney (University of Western Ontario).

I should also like to thank Gillian Nineham and her colleagues at Radcliffe Publishing for their encouragement to write this extended second edition.

In relation to the personal research work referred to at various points throughout the text I am indebted to a long list of individuals. However, I should like to express my particular gratitude to Mr Alan Rigby, statistician, and to Mrs Sara Mann, research administrator.

Finally, I should like to thank my family, Katrina, Ailie, Emily and Siân for their constant support and encouragement.

List of abbreviations

BNP	B-type natriuretic peptide
BMD	bone mineral density
CA-125	cancer antigen 125
CNS	central nervous system
COPD	chronic obstructive airways disease
CRP	C-reactive protein
CT	computed tomography
DEXA	dual energy X-ray absorptiometry
DVT	deep-vein thrombosis
ECG	electrocardiogram
ECHO	echocardiogram
EEG	electroencephalogram
ENT	ear, nose and throat
ESR	erythrocyte sedimentation rate
FSH	follicle-stimulating hormone
GGT	gamma glutamyl transferase
GI	gastro-intestinal
GP	general practitioner
HbA1c	glycated haemoglobin
INR	international normalised ratio
LR	likelihood ratio
LR+	positive likelihood ratio
LR−	negative likelihood ratio
MCV	mean cell volume
MRI	magnetic resonance imaging
NICE	National Institute for Health and Clinical Excellence
NSAID	non-steroidal anti-inflammatory drug
PE	pulmonary embolism
PSA	prostate-specific antigen
ROC	receiver operator characteristic

SiDPP   symptom-initiated diagnostic processing pathway
TB   tuberculosis
TIA   transient ischaemic attack
UTI   urinary tract infection

CHAPTER 1

Introduction

Two women, two breast lumps and two complaints provided me with an early insight into the difficulties of diagnosis in primary care. One patient subsequently grumbled that I had referred her on too quickly and caused her unwarranted distress. The other complained that I had responded too slowly and that the treatment of her cancer had been unnecessarily delayed. With hindsight, although the clinical findings in the two situations were virtually identical, I had clearly neglected to extract sufficient information from either patient about their respective concerns, nor had I established appropriate thresholds for further intervention.

Diagnosis has always been difficult. However, working as a primary care clinician it often seems to me that the development of new technologies coupled with the rising expectations of the public and the media have made the diagnostic process even more complex in recent years.

Nowadays it is easy to arrange a battery of investigations and, as a result, the traditional clinical encounter has changed, with much less focus on the patient as a person. In some situations the patient may barely have had the opportunity to say more than a few words before the clinician is arranging endoscopes, imaging or pathology/physiology testing. The simple clinical examination has also been downgraded: a patient of mine with a small leg ulcer recently came to see me quite distressed after a 'Doppler Assessment'. He had been informed that there was no blood flowing to his feet and that he required an urgent referral as his leg was at risk. Although palpating his foot pulses was surprisingly easy, it took me considerable time and effort (and another 'Doppler Assessment') to convince him that my clinical examination was correct. Equally worryingly I have encountered patients whose treatment has been delayed until they have been 'fully investigated'. I was once consulted by a patient who had been wheezing for 3 months with spirometry readings characteristic of asthma. The previous clinician involved had arranged for him to have a chest radiograph before commencing any specific treatment. Unfortunately as the patient had not felt well enough to travel the 20 miles to the radiology department, he had remained untreated and, for two months, had resorted to buying cough linctus from the local chemist.

Weight loss is a common symptom with a range of possible causes: 'organic' diseases such as cancer and thyroid dysfunction as well as 'non-organic' problems such as anxiety and depression. I can remember a patient with this symptom who had been extensively investigated by my local teaching hospital colleagues. She came into the surgery one day looking extremely low and, during the subsequent consultation, the question asked by my former boss was simple: 'Did you feel depressed before you went through all the tests?'. She burst into tears, 'I have always felt low but no one asked'. All her investigations were normal and she was subsequently successfully treated for her depression.

This book is about repositioning the patient back at the centre of the diagnostic process. In unravelling the significance of a symptom the patient can provide much of the diagnostic input and should also be more carefully considered and consulted about any subsequent investigations. Furthermore, the ultimate value of any diagnostic processing must be judged by its impact on the patient's wellbeing.

The diagnostic interaction between the patient and their doctor is not a passive process. Primary care diagnostics entails general practitioners developing an awareness of both the validity and the reliability of the clinical information provided by or obtained from patients and learning how to use it more rationally. In some cases a management decision can be made based only on the history, whereas in other situations the patient might need to be examined or appropriate investigations arranged. Diagnosis raises some awkward dilemmas about the appropriate use of new technologies and scientific evidence, the interface between diagnosis and screening together with doctors' abilities to make rational judgements in a situation of uncertainty.

Primary care diagnostics is also of relevance to those charged with commissioning diagnostic services. In a recent UK Department of Health press release highlighting the expansion in magnetic resonance imaging (MRI) the accompanying notes stated that MRI scans help 'diagnose … acute or chronic migraine and headaches'. However, headache is the most common symptom that patients bring to primary care clinicians and a large proportion of these seem to have no clear-cut explanation. In such circumstances, there is a significant risk that patients receive extensive and expensive investigations that are of limited value and potentially damaging physically and psychologically.

This book also represents a personal journey in which I have attempted to improve my own diagnostic skills with the assistance of clinical epidemiologists, psychologists, patients and clinical colleagues. I do not know whether I have achieved my objective; the only real certainty about attempting to make diagnoses in primary care is that I will continue to get it wrong sometimes!

CHAPTER 2

Diagnostic difficulties

INTRODUCTION

On Monday morning, I receive a telephone call from the consultant specialist congratulating me on my rapid referral of a patient with colorectal cancer. The patient, a middle-aged lady, had presented with a brief history of rectal bleeding, a slight change in bowel habit and an elevated erythrocyte sedimentation rate (ESR). Over the next few weeks, buoyed up by the consultant's praise and concerned not to damage my 'reputation', I referred a large number of similar patients and encouraged my colleagues to follow suit. However, the subsequent month a rather less complimentary letter arrived from the consultant indicating that I was 'clogging up his urgent clinics with a lot of dubious referrals'. I was rather bruised by this and immediately shifted to take up a more restricted referral practice in patients with rectal bleeding. Three months later I received an angry letter from a relative of a patient who had died of colorectal cancer, having been admitted as an emergency via casualty. According to the relative, the patient had previously consulted me with rectal bleeding but, although I had examined her, I had not initiated a referral. The letter went on to point out that 'according to the specialist all such patients should be referred and I had behaved recklessly'.

Although fictitious, the above scenario illustrates the unenviable position in which primary care clinicians are often placed. We have to balance often conflicting pressures using evidence and training which does not necessarily furnish us with sufficient skills to make a good judgement. Traditional teaching disseminated from specialist centres is focused on consultant encounters and the increasing use of new technologies. This educational programming is further underpinned by a natural tendency of specialists to judge our practice from their perspective. Thus, patients with symptoms of possible oncological significance who are encountered by primary care physicians will fall (over a period of time) into four groups.

1 Those who are referred on immediately and turn out to have significant disease (the 'good doctor').
2 Those who are initially missed and who reach the specialist later than ideal (the 'poor doctor').

3 Those who are referred but do not require specialist treatment (the 'overcautious doctor').
4 Those who are not referred and do not require specialist treatment (the 'gatekeeper role' of the primary care clinician).

Specialists who provide feedback to primary care physicians as well as clinical training for medical students obviously never encounter the vast majority of patients seen in primary care (group 4). Their educational activity is distorted towards addressing perceived inadequacies in groups 2 and 3. Unfortunately, there is often little appreciation that the information being promoted by such individuals may not assist primary care physicians in making a rational decision.

As a primary care clinician I have always found diagnosis particularly tricky due to its inherent uncertainty. It seems to me that to stop investigating a patient is often much more difficult than to start. When I order a colonoscopy for an individual with abdominal pain I sometimes wonder whose uncertainty I am managing and who will benefit most from the result. Hippocrates made an intriguing admission that one of the aims of diagnosis is to impress the patient and for a doctor to 'increase his reputation as a medical practitioner'.[1] Over the years I have encountered primary care physicians who have been labelled as 'astute' or even 'brilliant' diagnosticians but, on closer inspection, it seems that many of them are simply working at a different level of uncertainty than the rest of us. If an endoscopist perforates the bowel wall while undertaking a colonoscopy or if the patient suffers a myocardial infarction squashed in the MRI scanner, the primary care clinician can still claim that *they* did their best. The same argument used to apply to warfarinisation in patients with atrial fibrillation; a bleed in a patient given warfarin is the doctor's responsibility whereas a stroke in a patient not on warfarin was simply an 'act of God'. However, as patients gain more autonomy, such 'acts of God' are more carefully scrutinised.

Diagnosis highlights a number of difficulties, some of which will be considered in this chapter. However, one fundamental problem is the use of the term 'diagnosis'. In this book primary care diagnostics is defined as the rational collection *and use* of (additional) clinical information* (clinical indicants*) in the context of a known *abnormality* (e.g. a symptom, a sign or an incidental test finding) presenting to a primary care clinician with the intention of:

• detecting or excluding disorders by increasing the certainty as to their presence or absence, *and*
• contributing to the decision-making process with regard to further diagnostic and therapeutic management, *and*
• impacting on patient and health service outcomes.

See Glossary.

Patient-oriented outcomes include mortality, morbidity, disability, discomfort and satisfaction. Commissioners of diagnostic services will also be interested in, for example, enhanced efficiency, equity, accessibility and optimality (i.e. balancing improvements in health against the cost of such improvements).

INACCURACY AND INEFFICIENCY

Failing to recognise potentially serious illness in an accurate and efficient fashion can have adverse consequences for the delivery of high quality healthcare. Inaccuracy is about not identifying the true disease state, resulting in false-positive and false-negative diagnoses. The diagnosis may be missed, the diagnosis might be delayed or it may simply be incorrect. Inefficiency concerns the inappropriate or excessive use of tests or procedures beyond those needed to make a diagnosis in a timely and cost-effective manner.

Diagnostic errors or inefficiencies have certain consequences including the use of additional (and perhaps unnecessary, inappropriate or even harmful) services. Alternatively, there may be delays in the use of services until the condition has reached a more severe stage. Outcomes may be worse and costs higher with poorer patient or practitioner satisfaction and increased actions for malpractice.

For patients with cancer, false-negative diagnostic inaccuracies and inefficiencies can have adverse effects on prognosis as well as the nature of the interventions required. Randomised controlled trials of breast cancer and colorectal cancer screening have demonstrated significant effects on mortality as a consequence of detecting cancers earlier. In relation to symptomatic breast cancer patients Richards *et al.* demonstrated that delays of 3–6 months were associated with lower survival.[2]

Delayed cancer recognition as a result of inaccuracy or inefficiency may also lead to increases in patient distress and disability in addition to the eventual requirement for more radical therapies. For example, patients with late-stage testicular cancer or cutaneous melanoma need more extensive and aggressive treatment than those with early-stage disease.

Rheumatoid arthritis is another condition in which improvements in diagnosis (in terms of reductions in false-negatives) could have significant impacts on outcomes. The condition is now recognised to spread in a manner analogous to malignancy, increasing the synovial mass and involving new joints. Lard *et al.* observed a more favourable course among patients with rheumatoid arthritis who were treated with disease-modifying anti-rheumatic drugs early in their disease, when compared with patients who did not receive such medication until their disease course appeared to be persistently active.[3] Lard *et al.* suggested that early diagnosis and referral of patients with rheumatoid arthritis is crucial for optimal medical care. Furthermore, it has been proposed that early rheumatoid disease exhibits special immunological features making it a potential target for different therapeutic approaches.

It is always necessary to strike a sensible balance between under-diagnosis and over-diagnosis. The term 'diagnostic inaccuracy' also incorporates a consideration of false-positives, and such incorrect diagnoses may lead to inappropriate or even harmful investigation and treatment. For example, normal children who are misdiagnosed as having organic heart disease show as much deterioration in physical and social function as children who really do have damaged hearts.[4]

Concerns have also been expressed about false-positive diagnoses of common conditions such as heart failure or hypertension in adults. At least two studies have revealed that between one-third and two-thirds of patients may be receiving unnecessary drug treatment for heart failure.[5,6] In the case of hypertension there is evidence of increased absenteeism from work after diagnosis as well as negative effects on patients' perceptions of their ability to recover from unrelated acute illnesses.[7,8]

At a broader level, failure to make accurate and efficient diagnoses may have dramatic effects on health and social costs. The more intensive treatment required for advanced breast cancer increases direct medical care costs. Furthermore, significant indirect costs relate to the heightened pain and suffering in addition to the expense of lost productivity due to the shortened life expectancy. Another indirect cost of delayed diagnosis of breast cancer is awards from malpractice compensation claims. However, all these issues need to be balanced against similar costs arising from the adverse consequences of investigations.

To be effective diagnostic services should satisfy the following criteria:
- minimise the number of diagnoses completely missed
- minimise the number of delayed diagnoses that, in turn, retard appropriate therapeutic interventions with negative effects on patient outcomes
- minimise the number of incorrect diagnoses that may lead to inappropriate or even harmful treatment and unnecessary expenditure
- minimise the inappropriate or excessive use of investigations or procedures beyond those needed to make a diagnosis in a timely and cost-effective manner.

SCREENING AND SYMPTOMATIC DIAGNOSIS

In seeking to enhance the accuracy of diagnoses, a range of different interventions have been targeted both at patients and at healthcare professionals. Such approaches can be broadly divided into those focusing on population-based health screening and those designed to enhance the ability of primary care practitioners and patients to recognise and respond appropriately to symptoms or signs. However, in seeking to develop any solution to the problem of early diagnosis it is extremely important to consider the context in which the initiative has been developed and the setting where it will be applied.

Population-based screening is intuitively attractive, and often it is seen as the obvious first choice for earlier disease recognition. However, the real success of a screening programme is judged not by the ability of a new test to detect asymptomatic disease and improve patient survival under ideal conditions but rather to detect it with acceptable efficiency within the context of a community. In assessing the effectiveness of a screening programme, the effects of variations in subject compliance, administrative errors (e.g. incomplete and inaccurate patient lists) and laboratory/radiology deficiencies have to be taken into account. For example, there is little doubt that colorectal cancer screening using faecal occult blood has significant effects on mortality but in the Nottingham randomised controlled trial compliance rates were under 60%.[9] Screening for asymptomatic conditions is also not necessarily cheaper than responding appropriately to symptoms. In one economic analysis, it was demonstrated that the evaluation of the colon in people under the age of 50 with isolated rectal bleeding increased the life expectancy at a cost comparable to that of colon cancer screening.[10]

Screening is defined as the *'presumptive identification* of unrecognised disease or defects by the application of tests, examinations or other procedures that can be applied *rapidly'*. The use of the words 'presumptive' and 'rapid' emphasise that screening is merely the first stage in a process. In the UK, the government is now rolling out a national bowel-screening programme using faecal occult blood testing. However, concerns have been expressed that the UK NHS will not be able to cope with the number of extra colonoscopies needed as a result of the screening programme, a problem exacerbated by the fact that the test gives a high number of false-positive results. One major London hospital, for example, already has an average wait of 12 months for non-urgent colonoscopies. It is still not clear where such hospitals are going to find the staff to perform the extra investigations, nor how doctors can protect the interests of those patients who need colonoscopies but who are not in the screening programme.[11]

There are other concerns that screening targets interventions at asymptomatic members of the general public and everyone involved should fully appreciate the imperfections of all screening tests and the need for continuing vigilance for new symptoms. Unfortunately, some people may be falsely reassured and not understand the purposes of screening or the limitations of screening tests. The screening may even make the situation worse by causing patients to delay consulting their primary care physician about a possibly significant symptom.

Symptomatic approaches to earlier disease recognition by primary care practitioners differ from screening in that they are about risk assessment and rational judgements by doctors rather than risk reduction. It has also been suggested that as symptomatic diagnosis is 'patient initiated' as opposed to 'doctor initiated', the clinician has less responsibility to make the patient fully aware of the nature of the evidence. I take issue with this suggestion as some doctors seem to have interpreted it as a licence to use poorer evidence or to adopt a less patient-centred approach for diagnostics compared to screening.

In seeking to enhance the primary care physician's ability to recognise and appropriately respond to symptoms a plethora of educational initiatives, guidelines, and decision support tools have been developed in Europe, North America and Australasia. However, although few would argue against Howie's view[12] that symptomatic disease recognition is a core element of clinical primary care practice; beneath this broad consensus there is a major problem of applicability to the primary care context. Many such initiatives are built on clinical indicants derived from consultant encounters with partially ordered and highly selected groups of patients, a greater proportion of whom will have serious physical illness. Furthermore, the decision-making mechanisms being used are often insufficiently in tune with the realities of day-to-day primary care practice and our patients in terms of, for example, diagnostic precision and action thresholds.

There are a number of possible reasons why the primary care and patient perspectives have often been ignored in many of the centrally driven initiatives but it seems most likely that the problem represents an amalgam of educational tradition together with a lack of good quality, accessible diagnostic information applicable to the initial clinical encounter. In seeking to identify evidence to assist in diagnosis in primary care it seems that, in many areas, clinical research has not yet addressed in any meaningful manner what symptoms and signs indicate in primary care; just how useful is a particular symptom at predicting a disease, which symptoms are not useful, and which symptoms will rule out disease.[13]

The NICE *Referral Guidelines for Suspected Cancer* aimed at UK general practitioners serves as a good example of the problem.[14] The guidelines were developed in response to concerns that, if not properly managed, the UK government's decision to set a 2-week referral target for patients with suspected cancers would lead to a massive over-referral of patients with symptoms of possible oncological significance but no actual cancer. In an ideal world, the first step in developing any such guidance would be to undertake a systematic literature search in order to identify applicable evidence. Unfortunately, previous work had already suggested that the evidence base for symptomatic cancer diagnosis in relation to the initial clinical encounter (in low prevalence populations) was severely deficient.[15] Additionally, systematic reviews had revealed that there was a distinct lack of information concerning the significance of, for example, chronic cough as a feature of lung cancer or haematuria as a symptom of urological malignancy within primary care populations. Consequently, in the absence of clear-cut evidence, consensus adjustments were made in order to add weight to indicants and alter the thresholds for action. The outcome was the promotion of guidance that both ignored the primary care context and promoted a distorted version of secondary care-derived clinical evidence. This resulted in undesired effects on general practitioners' referral practices and outpatient capacity problems. Calls for the initiative to be scrapped have been prompted by a review of 35 studies, all of which found no evidence for any impacts on patient survival.[16] However, intriguingly, the perceived failure of the guidance for symptomatic lung cancer diagnosis has been cited as evidence in favour of lung cancer screening with spiral CT scanning rather than highlighting any inadequacies in the underlying evidence base (*see* Chapter 9).

USE OF TECHNOLOGY

It has long been claimed that a diagnosis could be achieved by history taking alone in the majority of patients. In order to evaluate the relative importance of the medical history, the physical examination and laboratory investigations in diagnosis a prospective study was undertaken of 80 patients attending four general medical outpatient departments in the UK.[17] Four different physicians were asked to record their diagnoses after taking the history and again after performing the physical examination. In 66 (83%) of the patients the medical history provided enough information to make an initial diagnosis of a specific disease entity which agreed with the one finally accepted. The physical examination was useful in making the diagnosis in only seven (9%) patients, though in 25 patients it served to change the physician's confidence in the diagnosis which he had already reached on the basis of the history. In a similar, but considerably larger study involving 630 medical outpatients, the history and the examination determined 56% and 17% of the diagnoses, respectively. Moreover, the findings suggested that across the whole of the UK in 1979, there was considerable wastage of resources (£3.5 million) as a result of unnecessary investigations.[18]

In the US, Peterson and colleagues have made similar findings, ascribing 76% of the diagnostic potential to the history and 12% to the clinical examination.[19] Furthermore, the importance of the history also applies to specific symptom groups such as patients presenting with dyspnoea, palpitations or dizziness. For example, Schmitt and colleagues compared the history-related diagnoses with the final diagnoses for patients admitted to hospital with dyspnoea. The history-based diagnoses accurately predicted the final diagnoses 74% of the time.[20]

Population-based studies provide some further indications that what happens to patients in the early symptomatic and low technology stages of the diagnostic process within primary care does matter in terms of their eventual outcome. Comparative studies across Europe have highlighted a potential for improvements in cancer recognition as assessed by the stage at patient presentation for definitive treatment. The pathway to care in patients with, for example, colorectal cancer is often very complex: in the absence of a screening programme it involves a combination of patient, professional and administrative reactions to symptoms of possible oncological significance. However, compared to the UK, it seems that primary care physicians in The Netherlands are receiving patients at an earlier Duke's stage with consequent improvements in survival.[21] Other evidence from a cross-sectional study in certain US states suggests that the primary care provision is important in earlier cancer diagnosis. Roetzheim *et al.* have demonstrated that the supply of primary care physicians is significantly correlated with the stage at diagnosis of patients with colorectal cancer: as the supply of primary care physicians increased, the odds of late-stage diagnosis decreased.[22]

In contrast to the increasing ambivalence about the use of the medical history and clinical examination, there seems to be a perception that diagnostic testing using the newer technologies is universally beneficial: this is not the case. A careful balance is required between risks and benefits in relation to the following areas:

- the adverse effects of technology
- the adverse effects of diagnostic delay
- psychological harms
- the impact on patient/health service finances.

Before primary care clinicians decide to undertake more complex investigations, there is always a need to appreciate that not every 'abnormality' is synonymous with organic disease and, for those that are, there may be no effective treatment. Kroenke *et al.* demonstrated that no specific physical disorder could be established as the cause in 30–75% of patients with symptoms, even after careful investigation.[23] Moreover, a large proportion of patients with one unexplained clinical condition such as fibromyalgia may meet the criteria for a second unexplained condition such as irritable bowel syndrome. Unfortunately the trend towards greater specialisation (and sub-specialisation) of doctors and technologies may push such individuals down a cascade of inappropriate diagnostic interventions and cross-referrals once they leave the holistic domain of the primary care physician.

Doctors in the US and Canada now order increasing numbers of cardiac investigations for patients, but with no significant effect on the incidence of acute myocardial infarction (a key outcome of interest in relation to possible cardiac symptoms).[24] It has been suggested that the growing costs of such health technology might threaten the Canadian health insurance system. Writing in the *American Journal of Medicine* in 1989 Kroenke *et al.* examined the costs incurred in the investigation of 12 common symptoms. They noted the very high price of discovering an organic diagnosis, amounting to $7778 for headache, $7263 for back pain and $4354 for chest pain.[23]

In the UK inadequate consideration is given to the integration of new technology into the diagnostic process with inconsistencies between commissioners in relation to application and purchasing. A particular concern is the lack of any coordination between high- and low-technology diagnostic approaches. Some commissioners may focus on purchasing high-technology machinery (e.g. MRI scans) and the infrastructure directly related to that equipment but ignore low-technology approaches such as blood tests or the doctor's clinical assessment. Aside from the possibility that low-technology interventions have a potentially greater impact on achieving a diagnosis, inadequacies in their use may have important knock-on effects on the use of the limited capacity high technology resources. There are also often difficulties with communication between, for example, primary care clinicians and radiologists. Poor clinical information provided by the former may impact on the quality of the feedback provided by the latter.

From the patient's perspective a related issue is that the drive towards increasing diagnostic capacity appears to have taken precedence over increasing diagnostic efficiency along the diagnostic processing pathway. Consideration is not always given to the integration of investigations within a single location, on a single day or by the means of mobile diagnostic units. Provision may also become inequitable if the equipment is inaccessible to some in terms of, for example, opening times or geographical location (*see* Chapter 10).

Technology and technological requirements are also continually changing and, for example, in developing services for patients with 'abdominal disorders', commissioners need to be aware of changes in equipment (e.g. virtual colonoscopy or the use of capsules), new diagnostic approaches (e.g. molecular and biological markers), a growing number of elderly patients with significant co-morbidities/co-treatments and changes in disease prevalence or treatment (e.g. in relation to irritable bowel or coeliac disease). Similarly, in the assessment of patients with low back pain, the advent of tumour necrosis factor inhibitors has highlighted the importance of seeking to diagnose ankylosing spondylitis at an earlier stage than was the case previously. The difficulty is how best to accommodate such changes and developments.

HEURISTICS AND BIASES

Diagnostics is about coping with uncertainty and we will always make mistakes. However, over-reliance on secondary care clinical experience or dogma by doctors working within primary care settings can result in key cognitive errors.

Some diagnoses, such as shingles or Down's syndrome, are simply about pattern recognition or spot diagnosis. Unfortunately the vast majority of patients do not conform to 'standard presentations' and, in most circumstances, it seems that primary care clinicians adopt a hypothetico-deductive approach to diagnosis. The initial step in this process involves the construction and the ranking of a provisional list of diagnostic possibilities. This requires the amalgamation of medical knowledge/experience and the patient's presenting complaint in relation to the primary care context, the patient's age/sex and any previous knowledge about that individual (the patient history), their family and their environment. Selective information gathering is then used to test the diagnostic hypotheses and subsequently to revise/re-rank the diagnostic list. This process of 'educated guessing' and testing is then repeated until a decision can be reached.

Unfortunately, it is now recognised that the capacity to carry out such a rational approach is, to some extent, limited or bounded by the size of an individual's working memory. As a result of this, decision making is often partially dependent on a number of cognitive heuristics or 'rules of thumb' in order to aid recall or to understand knowledge. A failure to appreciate that they may be using such heuristics can result in important mistakes being made by clinicians working in a primary care context who have spent a significant period employed or studying in secondary or tertiary care settings. For example, we may produce a distorted range of differential diagnoses through failing to take into account the relative prevalences of conditions in a primary care setting. This is an example of the 'representativeness heuristic' whereby we assume that something that seems similar to other things in a certain group is itself a member of that set. Unfortunately, in many situations the group membership is wrongly assigned. For example, when confronted with a 65-year-old man with chest pain I need to be aware that I am now sitting in a British general practice rather than a coronary care unit. Also the fact that men have more ischaemic heart disease than women does not mean that all men with chest pain have ischaemic heart disease.

Errors arising from inappropriate application of the representativeness heuristic may also impact on clinical features as well as on the diseases themselves. Some doctors may exhibit 'cue blindness' where they fail to respond to the information presented by the patient if it does not accord with their clinical experience. Kuyvenhoven *et al.* have noted that some general practitioners confronted by a patient with ambiguous symptoms may adopt a biased style in which the initial problem is inadequately defined and inappropriate diagnostic hypotheses are generated.[25]

'Confirmatory bias' is the related tendency to look for information that fits with our pre-existing expectations. In taking the medical history we might focus mainly on asking questions that simply confirm earlier judgements. As a result we may terminate the patient interview prematurely and fail to elicit some key information. Data that contradict our expectations also tends to be ignored or dismissed as unimportant, especially if they are obtained towards the end of the consultation. However, we are all well aware of the critical opportunities that occur when the patient is turning the door handle to leave the room and suddenly begins to outline their true reason for their visit. In relation to diagnosis it is very important to be aware of confirmatory bias and, after sighing and glancing at our watch (!), to give any new information careful consideration.

The situation is often further compounded by the 'availability heuristic' in which the probability of an event is judged by the ease with which it can be remembered. Availability in memory is affected by other characteristics of an event aside from its frequency, such as vividness, consequences for the physician or patient, recentness and rarity. In using this heuristic one particular problem faced by primary care practitioners is that they may not explicitly consider their own personal experience of the event within the population in which they are now working and/or attach undue significance to their small and unrepresentative experience with the disease. For example, the average full-time UK general practitioner will only encounter up to eight new cases of cancer per annum and hence most of their experience with new diagnoses will be derived from their time as a medical student or junior hospital doctor working in specialist settings. Currently I know that I am more likely to consider pulmonary embolus in the differential diagnosis of chest pain as I have just spotted one case and yet missed another.

A third heuristic, 'anchoring and adjustment', is the mental process whereby probability estimates are assigned. It involves specifying an initial estimate of risk (anchor) and arriving at a final estimate by making adjustments in the face of new information. Errors in relation to this heuristic are particularly important for primary care, as many of us tend to set the anchor incorrectly. Our initial probability estimates tend to be extreme – either too close to one or too close to zero. There is a particular tendency to overestimate the likelihood of events that are defined only if several characteristics all occur at once but to underestimate the likelihood if any one of several features occurs. Anchoring is something that will be touched on again in Chapter 3 in relation to Bayes' Theorem.

I know that sometimes I can be a little over-confident about my clinical skills. I have also worked with colleagues who would regularly make rapid 'barn-door' but incorrect diagnoses of, for example, thyrotoxicosis or papilloedema. Avoiding such over-confidence is not easy as much of my medical training seemed to emphasise a correlation between certainty and competence! Addressing over-confidence is about becoming more aware of the validity and the reliability of the diagnostic information that we might extract from patients in the context of the history and the examination. We must also avoid drawing false conclusions and deciding, erroneously, that two events (such as tiredness and anaemia in my case) are causally related whereas, in truth, it is all merely an illusion.

UNCERTAINTY

For primary care physicians diagnostic uncertainty is a particular problem as our knowledge is more general than specific, and patients consult us in the early and often undifferentiated stages of illness. In the presence of such uncertainty there is a need to be aware that we may respond to other pressures and alter treatment, investigation or referral thresholds based on considerations aside from the patient's clinical presentation.

The attitudes to risk taking in medical decision making have been studied amongst two groups of British and Dutch general practitioners. A number of statements were presented to the doctors in the form of a questionnaire, and the participants were asked to indicate their level of agreement with each one.[26] The results are shown in Table 2.1.

The results shown in Table 2.1 indicate that many doctors seek to minimise the risks that they are willing to take. Interestingly, when compared to their British counterparts, the Dutch doctors seemed better able to accommodate risk. Possible explanations for this may relate to differences in the system of medical education

TABLE 2.1 Levels of agreement with diagnostic statements by British and Dutch general practitioners

Statement	British GPs in agreement with statement (%)	Dutch GPs in agreement with statement (%)
When in doubt it is preferable to refer to a specialist than to wait and see	42	8
A GP must prefer the certain to the uncertain	32	20
A GP must not take any risks with physical illness	44	16
For physical complaints the GP should do everything possible to establish the cause of a complaint	65	25
As a GP you must always be aware that each complaint can be the beginning of a serious disease	88	47

and general practitioner training in The Netherlands. Having spent some time in Maastricht myself it does seem that there is a greater focus on teaching primary care physicians to be numerate in the belief that this may help them to deal better with uncertainty and low-level risk in the future.

In relation to diagnosis, physician uncertainty may also serve to devalue the history and the examination. Although the study by Peterson et al. referred to earlier[19] re-emphasised the particular value of the clinical history in achieving a diagnosis, the participating internists' diagnostic confidence increased from a ranking of 7.1 (on a scale of 1 to 10) after the history, to 8.2 after the physical examination and to as high as 9.3 after the laboratory investigations.

Positive defensive medicine is defined as the ordering of treatments, tests or procedures for the purpose of protecting the doctor from criticism rather than diagnosing or treating the patient. It has been suggested that diagnostic uncertainties within primary care is one of the key drivers in a shift towards positive defensive practice and the supply of care that is relatively unproductive for patients. In 1994, I conducted a national questionnaire survey of positive defensive medical practices by asking 500 UK doctors to answer 12 questions about the likelihood of specific practice changes in response to the possibility of a patient complaining.[27] Five years later the study was repeated using the same instrument and sampling frame (see Table 2.2).[28]

The results of both surveys indicate that doctors seem to have made significant practice changes as a result of the possibility of a patient complaining. Of the

TABLE 2.2 Positive defensive practice, 1994 and 1999

Positive defensive medical practice	% (No.) of practitioners stating likely or very likely to change		Odds ratios (and 95% confidence intervals) (compares 1994 and 1999)
	1994	1999	
Increased referral rate	63.8 (199)	72.7 (237)	1.51 (1.07–2.15)
Increased follow-up	63.4 (189)	68.4 (223)	1.19 (0.84–1.68)
Increased diagnostic testing	59.6 (177)	69.5 (228)	1.55 (1.10–2.18)
Consideration of diagnostic testing where there is a known element of risk	40.3 (116)	44.5 (143)	1.12 (0.80–1.58)
Prescription of unnecessary drugs	29.3 (87)	21.9 (71)	0.68 (0.49–1.00)

defensive medical practices adopted, the most common (over half of the doctors stating 'likely' or 'very likely') seemed to be increased diagnostic testing, increased referral rate and increased follow up. Over 30% of doctors often worried about being sued or having a complaint lodged against them and all the positive defensive medical practices were significantly associated with the practitioner's concerns about risk. The trends over the five years are also of some interest; in particular, in 1999, general practitioners stated that they were significantly more likely to undertake diagnostic testing or to refer patients than they had been five years previously.

In relation to primary care diagnostics, although some symptom-derived diagnostic pathways such as the approach to macroscopic haematuria or to haemoptysis are clear-cut, this is generally the exception. Symptoms such as tiredness and weight loss or abnormalities such as iron-deficiency anaemia raise awkward dilemmas about the management of uncertainty and the differential diagnosis of common problems. As a young, single-handed general practitioner I soon discovered that telling a patient with weight loss or fatigue that they might have depression was a remarkably efficient mechanism to get patients to leave my list! Nowadays I do better by explaining my diagnostic dilemma at the outset and yet making it quite clear that I am taking their problem seriously. I also find it quite helpful to outline any available information about the natural history and the likely prognosis of their symptom. For example, in relation to abdominal complaints unexplained after the initial history and the examination, over three-quarters resolve within a year.[29] With experience I have also moved away from a need to give everything an explanation or a label and patients seem to accept this. 'Your chest pain is not serious and is not from your heart and lungs but I am not sure about its exact cause; it may be muscular' seems to work better for me than simply stating that a pain is 'muscular'.

It is recognised that good communication between the doctor and their patient in a situation of uncertainty can have an important therapeutic role in managing symptoms. Moreover, work from Oregon and Colorado indicates that communication is correlated with malpractice claims. Compared with primary care physicians who had had a malpractice claim lodged against them, no-claims physicians used more statements of orientation (educating patients about what to expect) and tended to use more facilitation (soliciting patients' opinions, checking understanding and encouraging patients to talk).[30]

Unfortunately, policymakers also dislike diagnostic uncertainty and, in the UK, guidelines, non-doctor triage and access targets have been developed to seek to 'improve' matters. The problem of the evidence contained within some clinical guidance has been discussed earlier. However, a further concern is that once a guideline has been written and disseminated it may be adopted by those insufficiently trained or experienced to use it wisely and to be aware of its limitations (*see* Chapter 9).

Evidence-based practice represents an amalgam of good quality scientific research evidence in conjunction with clinical expertise and patient values. The role of the experienced primary care physician will always extend beyond the narrow application of other people's recommendations. Sullivan and MacNaughton have developed a helpful representation of the sources of evidence used during consultations (*see* Table 2.3).[31]

They further emphasise that *all* evidence should be carefully interpreted and individualised with the doctor 'acting wisely in the face of inevitable uncertainty'. In seeking to make a diagnosis and in applying any research evidence we must not lose sight of the subtle variations between patients in presentations of illnesses, understanding and acceptance of medical advice and treatment responses.

Although constructing a list of diagnostic hypotheses can be straightforward, imposing a hierarchy on the list and reaching a definite diagnostic conclusion is much trickier. Less skilled or experienced clinical staff may simply cope with

TABLE 2.3 Sources of evidence used during consultations[31]

Task	Undergraduate studies	Experience	Scientific evidence	Wider literature
Discover reason for patient's attendance	++	+++	+	++
Define clinical problem(s)	++	+++	+++	+
Address patient's concerns	++	+++	+++	++
Explain diagnosis to patient	+	+++	+	+++
Make effective use of consultation	+	+++	+++	+++

diagnostic uncertainty by using a 'diagnostic drag-net' that can easily result in the identification of other abnormal findings unrelated to the complaint presented by the patient. Rather than being reassured, both the clinician and the patient may then feel increasingly worried and a further series of tests or hospital referrals will inevitably follow. Discontinuity of care with the loss of the one responsible physician within primary care has also been shown to result in an increase in such inappropriate diagnostic testing. All this is compounded by the imperative to cut the time that a patient has to wait to access investigations.

Managing diagnostic uncertainty is very difficult but, as will be discussed further in subsequent chapters, in case of doubt it is well worth considering the use of time and a repeat consultation after an appropriate interval. The doctor also needs to be clear about his diagnostic strategy – is the purpose to rule in or to rule out a particular diagnosis? I would also support the suggestion from my Dutch colleagues of avoiding rushing to investigate complaints unexplained after taking an adequate history and conducting a competent clinical examination. They recommend waiting for at least 4 weeks after first presentation to the primary care physician as the probability that such a patient will be suffering from an, as yet, undetectable disease is very low. Furthermore, any initial investigations should be restricted to a full blood count, a blood glucose level, an ESR and a thyroid-stimulating hormone level measurement.[32]

Recently I received a brief note from a patient who had been to see me over several visits in relation to her 'dizziness'. The first consultation was quite awkward and difficult, the second was tricky but the last had been quite straightforward, as her problem had resolved. Managing uncertainty well and avoiding unnecessary (and potentially harmful) investigations and referrals can be very rewarding for both the doctor and the patient.

GENERAL REFERENCES

* Downie J, Elstein A, editors. *Professional Judgement: a reader in clinical decision making*. Cambridge: Cambridge University Press, 1988.
* Elstein AS, Schwarz A. Clinical problem solving and diagnostic decision making: selective review of the cognitive literature. *BMJ* 2002; **324**: 729–32.
* Gavin NI, Spock K, McNeill A, *et al. Diagnostic Accuracy in Primary Care: a review of the literature on five chronic conditions*. Rockville: Agency for Health Care Policy and Research, 1997.
* Heneghan C, Glasziou P, Thompson M, *et al.* Diagnostic strategies used in primary care. *BMJ* 2009; **338**: 1003–6.
* Jones R, Britten N, Culpepper L, *et al. Oxford Textbook of Primary Medical Care*. Oxford: Oxford University Press, 2003.
* Kramer BS, Gohagan JK, Prorok PC, editors. *Cancer screening: theory and practice*. New York: Marcel Dekker Inc., 1999.
* McWhinney IR. *A Textbook of Family Medicine*. Oxford: Oxford University Press, 1997.

- Sackett DL, Haynes RB, Guyatt GH, et al. *Clinical Epidemiology: a basic science for clinical medicine.* Boston: Little, Brown and Company, 1991.
- Tversky A, Kahneman D. Judgement under uncertainty: heuristics and biases. *Science* 1974; **185:** 1124–31.

TEXT REFERENCES

1. Hippocrates (Lloyd GER, editor). *Hippocratic Writings.* London: Penguin Books, 1978.
2. Richards MA, Westcombe AM, Love SB, et al. Influence of delay on survival in patients with breast cancer: a systematic review. *Lancet* 1999; **353:** 1119–26.
3. Lard LR, Visser H, Speyer I, et al. Early versus delayed treatment in patients with recent-onset rheumatoid arthritis: comparison of two cohorts who received different treatment strategies. *Am J Med* 2001; **111:** 446–51.
4. Bergman AB, Stamm SJ. The morbidity of cardiac non-disease in schoolchildren. *N Engl J Med* 1967; **276:** 1008–13.
5. Remes J, Miettinen H, Reunanen A, et al. Validity of clinical diagnosis of heart failure in primary healthcare. *European Heart Journal* 1991; **12:** 315–21.
6. Wheeldon NM, MacDonald TM, Flucker CJ, et al. Echocardiography in chronic heart failure in the community. *Quarterly Journal of Medicine* 1993; **86:** 17–23.
7. Mold JW, Hamm RM, Jafri B. The effect of labelling on perceived ability to recover from acute illnesses and injuries. *J Fam Pract* 2000; **49:** 437–40.
8. Haynes RB, Sackett DL, Taylor DW, et al. Increased absenteeism from work after detection and labelling of hypertensive patients. *N Engl J Med* 1978; **299:** 741–4.
9. Towler B, Irwig L, Glasziou P, et al. A systematic review of the effects of screening for colorectal cancer using the faecal occult blood test, Hemoccult. *BMJ* 1998; **317:** 559–65.
10. Lewis JD, Brown A, Localio R, et al. Initial evaluation of rectal bleeding in young persons: a cost-effectiveness analysis. *Ann Intern Med* 2002; **136:** 99–110.
11. Coombes R. Hanging in the balance. *BMJ* 2006; **332:** 384.
12. Howie JGR. Diagnosis – the Achilles' Heel? *J Roy Coll Gen Pract* 1972; **22:** 310–15.
13. Owen P. Clinical practice and medical research: bridging the divide between the two cultures. *Brit J Gen Pract* 1995; **45:** 557–60.
14. National Institute for Health and Clinical Excellence. *Referral Guidelines for Suspected Cancer.* London: NICE, 2005.
15. Summerton N. *Diagnosing Cancer in Primary Care.* Oxford: Radcliffe Medical Press, 1999.
16. Hanna SJ, Muneer A, Khalil KH. The 2-week wait for suspected cancer: time for a rethink? *Int J Clin Pract* 2005; **59:** 1334–45.
17. Hampton JR, Harrison MJG, Mitchell JRA. Relative contributions of history-taking, physical examination and laboratory investigation to diagnosis and management of medical outpatients. *BMJ* 1975; **2:** 486–9.
18. Sandler G. Costs of unnecessary tests. *BMJ* 1979; **2:** 21–4.
19. Peterson MC, Holbrook JH, Hales DV, et al. Contributions of the history, physical examination and laboratory investigation in making medical diagnoses. *West J Med* 1992; **156:** 163–5.
20. Schmitt BP, Kushner MS, Wiener SL. The diagnostic usefulness of the history in a patient with dyspnoea. *J Gen Intern Med* 1986; **1:** 386–93.

21. Gatta G, Capocaccia R, Sunt M, *et al.* Understanding variations in survival for color-ectal cancer in Europe: a EUROCARE high resolution study. *Gut* 2000; **47**: 533–8.

22. Roetzheim RG, Pal N, Gonzalez EC, *et al.* The effects of physician supply on the early detection of colorectal cancer. *J Fam Pract* 1999; **48**: 850–8.

23. Kroenke K, Mangelsdorff D. Common symptoms in ambulatory care. *Am J Med* 1989; **86**: 262–6.

24. Tanne JH. Heart disease tests increase, but attack rate is unchanged. *BMJ* 2006; **332**: 257.

25. Kuyvenhoven MM, Spreeuwenberg C, Touw-Otten FWMM. Diagnostic styles of general practitioners confronted with ambiguous symptoms. *Scand J Prim Health Care* 1989; **7**: 43–8.

26. Grol R, Whitfield M, De Maeseneer J, *et al.* Attitudes to risk taking in medical decision making among British, Dutch and Belgian general practitioners. *Brit J Gen Pract* 1990; **40**: 134–6.

27. Summerton N. Positive and negative factors in defensive medicine: a questionnaire study of general practitioners. *BMJ* 1995; **310**: 27–9.

28. Summerton N. Trends in negative defensive medicine within general practice. *Brit J Gen Pract* 2000; **50**: 565–6.

29. Kroenke K, Jackson JL. Outcome in general medical patients presenting with common symptoms: a prospective study with a 2-week and a 3-month follow-up. *Family Practice* 1998; **15**: 398–403.

30. Levinson W, Roter DL, Mullooly, *et al.* Physician-patient communication. The relationship with malpractice claims among primary care physicians and surgeons. *JAMA* 1997; **277**: 553–9.

31. Sullivan FM, MacNaughton RJ. Evidence in consultations: interpreted and individualised. *Lancet* 1996; **348**: 941–3.

32. Dinant GJ. NHG-Standard Bloedonderzoek. *Huisartsen Wetenschap* 1994; **37**: 202–11.

CHAPTER 3

Principles of primary care diagnostics

INTRODUCTION

Primary care diagnostics is about repositioning the patient and their interaction with the primary care physician back at the heart of the diagnostic process. The patient can provide much of the diagnostic input and, as discussed in Chapter 2, they have the potential to provide the majority of the information leading to a solution rather than simply be seen as presenting the problem. Patients should also be more carefully considered and consulted about the diagnostic approach and the outputs from the process.

As a primary care physician, whether I am interviewing or examining a patient, deciding if I should organise radiological or biochemical tests, commissioning diagnostic services or undertaking diagnostic research, a primary care approach should be adopted. The requirement is simply to place the emphasis on the patient as opposed to the disease, the available technology or the values and views of hospital-based specialists.

THE DIAGNOSTIC APPROACH

By focusing on the technology rather than the patient, there is often a failure to appreciate that, in most circumstances diagnosis involves a carefully specified sequence of actions rather than a single investigation. Moreover, important clinical information can be obtained from a careful assessment of a patient's symptoms, their past medical history, and the clinical examination in addition to biochemical, pathological, physiological and radiological tests. Diagnosis also sometimes involves simply observing patients over a period of time possibly combined with stopping or starting a treatment.

Primary care is defined as the setting where the first interaction takes place between a patient and a healthcare professional and represents the beginning (and often also the middle and the end) of the diagnostic processing pathway. It is important to appreciate that a number of pathways may originate from the same initiating abnormality; for example chronic cough can indicate a chest, ear/nose/throat, gastrointestinal, cardiac, iatrogenic or neurological problem. On the other hand an individual patient (especially if elderly and/or with significant co-morbidities) may sometimes present with more than one diagnostic dilemma.

General practitioners, family practitioners and other primary care clinicians encounter a much broader range of problems, many of which are presented in an undifferentiated fashion. Partially as a result of this, decisions made by primary care clinicians are dissimilar from those made by specialists – the precise diagnostic labels are often less important than deciding on an appropriate course of action. In primary care, diagnoses may be framed in terms of dichotomous decisions: treatment versus non-treatment, referral versus non-referral, and serious versus non-serious. In a general practice-based study of respiratory illness Howie concluded that a specific diagnostic label might be merely a justification for antibiotic treatment rather than a reason for it.[1] McWhinney emphasises the importance of eliminative diagnosis (the diagnosis of 'wellness') in addition to the observation that many illnesses in primary care defy any rigid diagnostic classification. For example, they can be transient or self-limiting or, in other circumstances, treated before they reach the stage of classical features revealing themselves.

The clinical information required to distinguish between, for example, two courses of action in a low-prevalence primary care population is different from that necessary to make a precise clinical diagnosis in a specialist setting. In keeping with this, when family physicians and general internists were confronted with the same simulated patient problems, the family physicians ordered fewer tests and offered a less precise diagnosis than did the specialists.[2] Broader approaches such as the use of non-specific investigations (e.g. erythrocyte sedimentation rate, plasma viscosity or C-reactive protein) may therefore be more appropriate to primary care decision making. Fraser contends that the medical history is particularly relevant to diagnosis in a situation where there are multiple, undifferentiated symptoms, often with a paucity of accompanying physical signs and the frequent absence of disease. However, in utilising symptoms it is necessary to distinguish between those symptoms that cause a patient to consult with their primary care clinician (iatrotropic) and those that are elicited during the course of the medical interview (non-iatrotropic).

THE PATIENT AS THE DIAGNOSTIC INPUT

Diagnostic processing commences when a patient presents with a *known* abnormality such as a symptom, a sign or an incidental test finding to a primary care physician. Moreover, the primary care clinician often already has access to key information about the patient such as their past medical history, family history, occupation and social circumstances. Unfortunately, as was discussed in Chapter 2, much of the interpretation placed on the primary care assessment is derived from experience of selected patients encountered in hospital settings.

Primary care diagnostics is about re-emphasising the importance of the primary-care based clinical encounter in the diagnostic process. Historically doctors would engage all their senses in extracting as much diagnostic information as possible from the patient. In *Epidemics* Hippocrates wrote 'we must consider the patient... his speech, his mannerisms, his silences, his habits of sleep or wakefulness... his stools, urine, sputum and vomit. Observe too sweating, shivering, chill, cough, sneezing, hiccough, the kind of breathing. We must determine the significance of all these signs'.[3] Although it would no longer seem appropriate to suggest a return to tasting urine for sugar, there seems no reason why we should neglect the other sensory inputs derived from hearing, seeing, touching and even smelling patients.

We can listen to the patient and to their relatives in addition to auscultating various body sounds. We can observe the patient in the waiting room, during the course of the consultation as well as in their home environment. We can also specifically look at skin rashes, moles, conjunctivae and sclerae.

Although all clinicians are familiar with the key elements of the clinical examination it is important to appreciate that some initial sensory data can be obtained when we first shake the patient's hand. Smell is also an underrated sense and, according to Bomback, much more information can be obtained this way than simply identifying smokers (or passive smokers). He points out that, in a closed consulting room, odours are much easier to appreciate than carotid bruits.[4] A patient complaining of a smelly vaginal discharge is more likely to have bacterial vaginosis than candidiasis.[5] Intriguingly it seems that dogs can even sniff out cancer possibly via some alterations in human leucocyte antigens, which determine some body odours.[6]

The primary care approach also appreciates that patients do not represent an empty vessel into which a symptom or sign appears; they also bring into the encounter values and expectations derived from their social circumstances and psychological state. They will have their own diagnostic concerns and understandings of risk which may not necessarily match those of their doctor. Consequently, although information obtained directly from the patient can represent powerful and easily accessible diagnostic input, there is a need to be aware of the limitations of such findings. Primary care clinicians using data supplied by or extracted from patients must give very careful consideration to the validity and the reliability of such information.

Validity of data

Validity is an assessment of the degree to which an item of clinical information relates to the 'truth' and one of the difficulties of using any such information is that it always exhibits less than perfect validity. In relation to enhancing primary care diagnosis there are three key elements to this 'truth':

- face validity
- predictive validity
- concurrent validity.

Face validity

Face validity is a subjective assessment as to whether an item of clinical information represents a reasonable diagnostic tool. Thus enquiries about rectal bleeding or haemoptysis appear to be broadly satisfactory questions to ask in relation to the diagnosis of colorectal or lung cancer respectively. However, seeking information on these same symptoms is not of obvious relevance (i.e. lacks face validity) in assessing a women's menopausal status.

There is a further issue to consider for face validity in relation to the clinical question that we are seeking to address. The most common clinical questions are listed in Table 3.1.

One of the problems of some clinical information is that it may be used to address more than one purpose and this can lead to confusion. For example, data derived from taking a family history or from faecal occult blood measurement may be used both for diagnosis and for screening. Dyspnoea, ankle swelling and B-type natriuretic peptide (BNP) might be used not only to assist in heart failure diagnosis, but also for risk/treatment stratification and to assess treatment response. In relation to cancer, symptoms have roles in initial diagnosis, diagnosis of recurrence and even for assessing prognosis.

Thus in using any so-called diagnostic data it is very important to be quite clear about their precise role in the context where they will be used. In particular are they *actually designed* to seek to make a diagnosis, or to guide therapy, or to assess prognosis, or to screen for unrecognised disease? Specific problems often occur at the interface between diagnosis (risk assessment) and screening (risk reduction). It is suggested that some screening tests are being inappropriately used for diagnostic purposes and some diagnostic tests are being used wrongly for screening. For

TABLE 3.1 Clinical questions

Issue	Question
Abnormality	Is the patient sick or well?
Diagnosis	Does the patient have a particular disease?
Frequency	How often does a particular disease occur?
Prognosis	What are the consequences of having a particular disease?
Treatment (including stratification and monitoring)	How does treatment change the course of a particular disease?
Prevention (including screening and risk stratification)	Does an intervention on well people keep a particular disease from arising? Does early detection and treatment improve the course of a particular disease?
Cause	What conditions lead to a particular disease? What are the pathogenetic mechanisms of a particular disease?
Cost	How much will care for an illness cost?

example, cytological examination of cervical smears has detection rather than diagnostic accuracy.[7] Thus a negative cytology report does not exclude cervical cancer and can simply cause delays or provide false reassurance. Conversely, liver function testing is not a recognised screening test and, although ordering such a test is easy, addressing the slight abnormalities that are often picked up can be extremely tricky and costly. Is the finding simply a statistical aberration? Should I repeat it? Should I refer for an opinion? Should I arrange further tests such as a liver ultrasound? I have certainly encountered patients who have ended up having a 'normal' liver biopsy (a procedure not without risk) as a consequence of an ill-considered tick on a biochemistry request form.

Predictive validity

Predictive validity represents the ability of the clinical information obtained at the patient encounter within primary care to predict the eventual outcome of interest (e.g. cancer, heart failure or depression).

Misunderstandings about the impact of symptom or disease prevalence and evolution on the predictive validity of an item of clinical information has led to fundamental disagreements between primary care clinicians and specialists regarding the usefulness of all types of clinical indicant. This seems to be particularly the case in relation to earlier cancer diagnosis where the majority of textbooks and guidelines appear to assume that such information can simply be transposed directly from studies amongst hospital patients to patients encountered in primary care. As is discussed in Chapters 8 and 9, much more diagnostic research should be focused towards assessing whether an item of clinical information (e.g. a symptom, a sign or a laboratory test result) is a valid indicator of, for example, colorectal cancer amongst patients presenting to primary care clinicians.

The predictive validity of any clinical indicant can be expressed in a number of ways – i.e. positive predictive value, sensitivity, specificity, likelihood ratio and receiver operator characteristic (ROC) curve. The definitions of these terms are given in Table 3.2.

The positive predictive value often makes the most intuitive sense to physicians. However, for the primary care clinician it is important to be aware that the predictive value is affected by the prevalence: as the prevalence falls, the number of false positives tends to increase resulting in a lowering of the positive predictive value (*see* Figure 3.1). A clinical indicant with 90% sensitivity and 95% specificity has a positive predictive value of 95% if the underlying prevalence of disease is 50%, but only 15% if the prevalence is 1%.

Traditionally sensitivities and specificities have been applied to laboratory testing but the functions can clearly be used to indicate the predictive validity of any type of clinical information. Sackett *et al.* have even developed the 'rules' SpPin and SnNout to make the terms more meaningful and useful for clinicians. The rule of SnNout states that if a clinical indicant has sufficiently high sensitivity, a negative

TABLE 3.2 Common measures of predictive validity

Measures of predictive validity	Definitions
Positive predictive value	The probability that the disease is present if the clinical indicant is positive [present] (the negative predictive value is the probability that the disease is absent if the clinical indicant is negative [absent]).
Sensitivity	The probability of a positive result in relation to the clinical information if the disease is present (the 'true-positive' rate).
Specificity	The probability of a negative result in relation to the clinical information if the disease is absent (the 'true-negative' rate).
Likelihood ratio	The likelihood that a given result in relation to the clinical information would be expected in a patient with the disease compared to the likelihood that the same result would be expected in a patient without the disease. Likelihood ratios indicate how many times more (or less) likely a result is in a patient with the disease compared to a patient free of disease.
Receiver operator characteristic (ROC) curve	A graphic representation of the relationship between the true-positive rate of a clinical indicant and the false-positive rate of the same clinical indicant as the criterion (cut-off point) of a positive result is changed.

result rules out the target disorder (i.e. less likely to be a false negative). The associated rule of SpPin states that if a clinical indicant has sufficiently high specificity, a positive result rules in the disorder (i.e. less likely to be a false positive). However, as a primary care clinician I am yet to identify a clinical indicant with sufficiently high sensitivity or specificity that would enable me to confidently apply either of these two 'rules'. It would also seem more sensible to consider the two measures together as they are clearly complementary. There is generally a requirement to make a trade

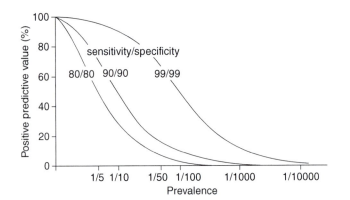

FIGURE 3.1 Positive predictive value according to sensitivity, specificity and prevalence of disease

off between sensitivity and specificity in deciding the cut-off point at which a clinical indicant represents a positive result. Such cut-off points are dependent on the setting and whether the purpose of the clinical indicant is to exclude or to confirm disease.

Unlike the predictive value, it is often assumed that the values for the sensitivity and specificity are fixed. This is not the case: the values for sensitivity and specificity are derived from studies in which the clinical information is compared against some reference standard approximating to the 'truth'. Unfortunately, the majority of such studies have been conducted in specialist settings and primary care clinicians need to know the nature of the study population if they are going to give meaning to the sensitivity and specificity values. There may also be a tendency to recruit cohorts of either healthy, self-selected volunteers such as medical students or less well populations from outpatient clinics into such studies. This is important as clinical information may only be positive (present) in extensive/advanced disease or in less well patients but negative (absent) in localised disease or in situations where there are significant co-morbidities. In registered general practice populations in The Netherlands, the prevalence of multimorbidity (two or more diseases at the same time) occurs in 29.7% of subjects, the prevalence increasing with age.[8]

Patients first presenting to primary care clinicians at the beginning of the diagnostic processing pathway will generally have conditions that are at an evolutionary stage when sensitivities and specificities of clinical indicants are changing. As time passes the characteristics of the clinical indicant may become fixed and moreover the patient will have had time to reflect on their story. Melbye *et al.* examined the value of reported dyspnoea, reported chest pain, chest crackles, temperature, ESR and C-reactive protein in relation to the diagnosis of pneumonia. They noted that illness duration had important effects on the predictive ability of these clinical indicants.[9]

In recent years there has been an increasing interest in the use of the 'likelihood ratio', which is a ratio between sensitivity and specificity. The magnitude of the likelihood ratio provides a measure of the predictive ability of the clinical indicant. Clinical indicants with likelihood ratios greater than one increase the chances of disease; the larger the likelihood ratio the more compelling the argument for disease. Conversely, clinical indicants that have likelihood ratios between one and zero decrease the probability of disease; the closer the likelihood ratio to zero, the more convincing the finding argues against disease. Some clinical findings, when present, have a dramatic effect on the likelihood of disease but change the probability little when they are absent. Other features are more useful if they are absent because the negative finding practically excludes disease.

The adjectives 'positive' or 'negative' indicate whether the likelihood ratio refers to the presence of the clinical information (positive) or the absence of the clinical information (negative). Positive likelihood ratios with the highest value argue most *for* disease when the clinical information is present (i.e. how the probability changes when the finding is present); negative likelihood ratios with the value closest to zero argue the most *against* disease when that clinical information is absent (i.e. how the probability changes when the finding is absent).

likelihood ratio*

$$= \frac{\text{proportion of patients } \textit{with} \text{ disease and } \textit{with} \text{ clinical finding}}{\text{proportion of patients } \textit{without} \text{ disease and } \textit{with} \text{ clinical finding}}$$

positive likelihood ratio*

$$= \frac{\text{proportion of patients } \textit{with} \text{ disease and } \textit{with} \text{ positive clinical finding}}{\text{proportion of patients } \textit{without} \text{ disease and } \textit{with} \text{ positive clinical finding}}$$

negative likelihood ratio*

$$= \frac{\text{proportion of patients } \textit{with} \text{ disease and } \textit{with} \text{ negative clinical finding}}{\text{proportion of patients } \textit{without} \text{ disease and } \textit{with} \text{ negative clinical finding}}$$

A particular advantage of using likelihood ratios as opposed to individual sensitivity and specificity values is that the characteristics of the clinical indicant can be combined into a single number. It is also possible to describe the indicant in a more clinically meaningful series of strata for different levels of the clinical finding. The use of likelihood ratios also avoids any major concerns about the possible impact of disease prevalence on the predictive validity. However, as in the case of all of the measures of predictive validity, likelihood ratios cannot be easily transposed from one population to another. The practical application of likelihood ratios will be discussed in greater detail in Chapters 5 and 6.

A pyramid can be used to illustrate the overall predictive validity problem to consider in relation to primary care diagnosis (*see* Figure 3.2). It has different levels representing the community, primary care, secondary care and tertiary care and the central shaded bar indicates patients with symptoms who turn out to have disease.

As patients ascend though the pyramid changes occur in the population cross-section at each level. For example, the positive predictive value of isolated rectal bleeding for colorectal cancer is less than 0.1% in the general population but 36% amongst patients subsequently reaching secondary care.[10] These differences in the patient spectrum at each level are dependent on the broad range of factors affecting both consultation and referral behaviour (e.g. the effects of demographics, co-morbidities, social circumstances and psychological variables) as well as the developments occurring because of the simple passage of time. Some symptoms will have a greater propensity to cause patients to consult and hence there may be little difference between the community and the primary care populations. Similarly some symptoms presenting to primary care clinicians might initiate an immediate

---

See Glossary.

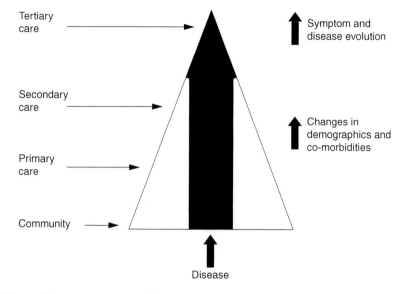

FIGURE 3.2 The symptom pyramid

referral. However, in the case of new-onset rectal bleeding, the factors affecting consultation and referral practices are multifactorial and remain only partially understood. It seems that colorectal cancer patients with significant co-morbidities are often referred on at an earlier pathological stage,[11] whereas older patients with symptoms suggestive of colorectal cancer are more likely to be admitted as emergencies with advanced disease[12] (*see* Chapter 9).

Furthermore, in a community setting the colorectal cancer will not only be at an earlier pathological stage, but other 'traditional' symptoms and signs (e.g. change in bowel habit, abdominal pain, weight loss) will also be less defined and developed.

Thus in assessing the predictive validity of the information provided by the patient to a primary care clinician there is a need to tread carefully. As I illustrate in Chapters 5 and 6, although likelihood ratios can easily be harnessed to assist in rational decision making, the origins of such numerical measures must to be very carefully considered. To practise primary care diagnostics there is a requirement to be confident that the discriminant information available to assist clinicians in assessing the predictive validity of the patient's initial story is actually applicable to the primary-care-based encounter.

Concurrent validity

Concurrent validity assesses the degree of mismatch between, for example, the patient's report about their symptoms or their past healthcare history and an appropriate reference standard (e.g. information obtained from other sources such as registries or relatives).

In relation to symptoms, a variety of factors may impact on the concurrent validity concerning the information, the interviewee (i.e. the patient) and the interviewer (i.e. the clinician). For example, although rectal bleeding/change in bowel habit may exhibit reasonable face and predictive validity for colorectal cancer diagnosis there may still be some worries about concurrent validity, i.e. how valid is the patient in stating they have (or have not) observed rectal bleeding in relation to them actually having rectal bleeding? The patient may never look at their motions or the design and colour of the toilet pan may make such observation difficult. Other patients might have poor vision (especially in a dimly lit cloakroom) or simply be colour blind.

Many issues relating to concurrent validity will be discussed in subsequent chapters but it is worth outlining here the four general ways in which interviews by primary care clinicians can lead to this problem.

1 **Asking errors** – For example, omitting questions or asking confusing or complicated questions. Answering the question 'have you seen the doctor recently?' depends on the patient's interpretation of the term 'recently'.
2 **Probing errors** – Probes are additional questions asked or statements made by the interviewer when the answer given by the patient is incomplete or irrelevant. However, we may fail to probe when necessary, our probing may be biased or irrelevant, or we may prevent the respondent from saying all that they wish to say.
3 **Recording errors** – For example, recording something not said, not recording something said, incorrectly recording what was said.
4 **Flagrant cheating** – For example, recording a response when a question is not asked or answered.

Reliability

There are two types of reliability that are of particular interest in practising primary care diagnostics: patient intra-observer reliability and doctor inter-observer reliability.

Patient reliability

Securing a reproducible response from a patient if the same question is asked two to three weeks apart is important if we are going to have confidence that an item of clinical information represents a useful diagnostic tool. Such intra-observer reliability will be considered further in relation to symptoms and the medical history in Chapters 4 and 5.

The most straightforward way to express intra-observer agreement is by simply calculating the proportion of agreement, but this ignores the effect of chance accounting for the findings. To assess the chance-corrected proportional agreement the kappa statistic is used and different ranges for kappa have been categorised with respect to the degree of agreement they suggest. Values greater than 0.80 may be taken to represent almost perfect agreement, values between 0.61 and 0.80 substantial agreement, values between 0.41 and 0.60 moderate agreement, values between 0.21 and 0.40 slight agreement and values of 0.20 or below represent poor agreement beyond chance.[13]

Doctor reliability

Ensuring that different doctors confronted with the same patient elicit similar information from the history or from the clinical examination is termed inter-observer reliability. It can also be assessed by the kappa statistic and this is considered further in Chapter 6.

It is important to appreciate that doctor inter-observer reliability is also influenced by the clinical context. For example, a combination of urinary symptoms, prostate nodularity with gross enlargement, age and prostate-specific antigen (PSA) might possibly be helpful to the primary care physician in differentiating between patients with or without potentially significant disease for onward referral. However, from the secondary care perspective, prostate nodularity with gross enlargement may well be a useless sign as all patients will have it (or else they would not have been referred!). The specialist may therefore be more concerned with, perhaps, the midline furrow or the fixation of the gland. However, it would clearly be wrong for the consultant to encourage the primary care clinician to switch over to use such findings in their decision making, as not only is the patient population different, but such 'detailed' findings are also likely to exhibit considerably lower levels of inter-observer reliability when used by generalists in primary care.

Diagnostic processing

In addition to re-focusing on the patient as a source of important diagnostic data, primary care diagnostics is also about seeking to exploit all diagnostic information (whether from the history, the examination or by means of investigations) in a more appropriate and rational fashion in the context of the diagnostic processing pathway. There is a requirement for doctors, patients and health managers to be aware of the limitations of even the most complex investigations in terms of false negatives and false positives. Furthermore, diagnosis should not be viewed as assimilating masses of information from tests in order to detect or exclude a disorder. There is a need to be confident that any investigation is only used after a careful consideration of the costs and consequences for the individual patient, their family and the healthcare budget. Some of these issues can be addressed by adopting a Bayesian approach, considering decision-making thresholds and risk communication and making better use of time. We also need to think very carefully before binding ourselves to any particular clinical decision rule or tool.

Adopting a Bayesian approach

Bayes' Theorem* is a very helpful tool to assist in both the understanding and the practice of primary care-oriented diagnostic processing by placing the likelihood ratios discussed earlier into a context. It is most clearly expressed in the form:

$$\text{posterior odds} = \text{likelihood ratio} \times \text{prior odds}$$

This formula emphasises that the interpretation of the significance of any new information should depend on our existing knowledge about the probability of a disease (the prior probability* or prior odds* of disease). Thus a patient who comes to see their primary care physician about a cough will already have a prior (existing) probability of lung cancer. This probability will be modified by additional information derived from the medical history to arrive at a new (post-history) probability of cancer. This probability may, in turn, be further adjusted by data derived from the clinical examination to produce a post-examination probability that, after a radiograph, could then become a post-test probability. Thus, in an idealised form, the diagnostic processing pathway can be seen as a number of probability steps increasing the certainty of disease (or absence of disease).

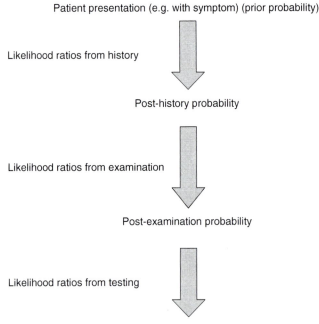

Patient presentation (e.g. with symptom) (prior probability)

Likelihood ratios from history

Post-history probability

Likelihood ratios from examination

Post-examination probability

Likelihood ratios from testing

Post-test probability (posterior probability)

It is important to be as confident as possible about the prior probability as this will clearly have a major impact on the posterior probability. For example Sox *et al.*

See Glossary.

compared the prevalence of coronary heart disease in patients who had similar histories but who came from populations with different disease prevalences (i.e. different prior probabilities).[14] They were able to demonstrate that the prevalence of coronary artery disease was much reduced in two primary care populations than in a referred arteriography population, even when patients with similar clinical histories were compared. Thus the general principle to emphasise is that, at the first clinical encounter in primary care, the posterior probability of disease will be lower than in a selected hospital population even if the same clinical indicants with identical likelihood ratios could be applied.

The importance of identifying applicable diagnostic likelihood ratios was touched on in the previous section and is considered further in Chapter 8. In relation to primary care-oriented diagnostic processing the additional problem of identifying prior probabilities also needs to be taken into account. Currently many such prior probabilities are derived from our own clinical experience but, as discussed in the previous chapter, we may be biased in the way this 'anchor' is set. Prevalence statistics have been used as a substitute but, unfortunately, they generally provide information on the probability of diseases in the general population or in some age/sex subset at a point before the patient actually comes to see the primary care clinician. What is really required to practise primary care diagnostics is data on the probability of disease amongst patients presenting with particular symptoms. Until recently this information was sparse and often relied on data derived from patients with symptoms studied in hospital outpatient departments, open access clinics or accident and emergency departments. Although the prior probability of myocardial infarction amongst patients presenting to an emergency room with acute chest is said to be 15%, certain selective factors will have already altered the make up of this population in comparison with patients with acute chest pain encountered by primary care clinicians.

Between 1985 and 1995 a group of 54 Dutch family physicians collected information on consultations in order to begin to develop a prior probability database for four common symptoms; cough, shortness of breath, general weakness/tiredness and lower back symptoms.[15] Some of the information on shortness of breath and general weakness/tiredness is shown in Tables 3.3 and 3.4.

In using such data in clinical practice, care should to be taken in relation to the validity of the final diagnoses and there is also a need to be aware of possible biases arising from both misclassifications and selective recording by participating clinicians. The critical evaluation of studies seeking to develop information on prior probabilities or likelihood ratios for patient-centred diagnosis within primary care is something that is considered further in Chapter 8.

Aside from being aware about the significance of the prior probability it is also important to appreciate that any linkage between the individual items of clinical information (i.e. their likelihood ratios) and the putative disease will be considerably weaker in a primary care than in a specialist setting. Thus, although a lower

TABLE 3.3 Prior probabilities for patients presenting with shortness of breath

Diagnosis	Prior probabilities (age 15–24 years) (%)	Prior probabilities (age 65–74 years) (%)
Acute bronchitis	18.1	33.5
Asthma	23.5	5.4
Heart failure	–	12.6
Hyperventilation	18.8	5.9
Head cold	8.1	3.0
Pneumonia	–	2.6
COPD/emphysema	–	5.2
Ischaemic heart disease	–	2.6
Viral disease	–	1.3
Chronic bronchitis/bronchiectasis	–	2.6
Atrial fibrillation/flutter	–	2.4
Adverse effect of medical agent in proper dose	–	1.5

level of disease-oriented diagnostic precision may be appropriate in primary care, this must be balanced against an ability to actually be able to make some kind of diagnostic decision.

Figure 3.3 illustrates how the prior (pre-test) probability relates to the posterior (post-test) probability according to different levels of likelihood ratios. This serves to demonstrate that clinical information is diagnostically more useful when the

TABLE 3.4 Prior probabilities for patients presenting with general weakness/tiredness

Diagnosis	Prior probabilities (age 15–24 years) (%)	Prior probabilities (age 65–74 years) (%)
Viral disease	8.0	8.0
Head cold	3.6	4.2
Iron-deficiency anaemia	4.4	2.4
Acute bronchitis	1.1	2.4
Adverse effect of medical agent in proper dose	1.1	4.2
Depressive disorder/feeling depressed	0.8	4.7
Other mental disorder	3.4	–
Influenza (proven)	1.7	2.3
Anxiety/stress	3.1	2.8
Infectious mononucleosis	3.2	–

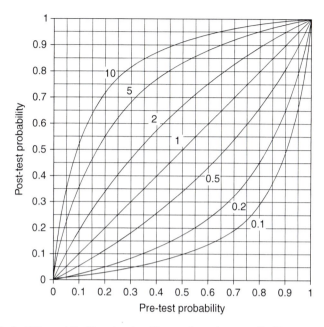

FIGURE 3.3 Probability and likelihood ratios (Curves for only seven likelihood ratios are shown.)

prior probabilities are between 20–80%, because in this range there is the greatest divergence of the likelihood ratio curves. Thus any likelihood ratios applied at the level of the clinical examination or investigations will have a much greater diagnostic impact if the input from the patient in the context of the medical history can be maximised (i.e. to enhance the magnitude of the post-history probability). Some example calculations are also detailed in Table 3.5.

To further strengthen an association between clinical information and diseases, combinations of clinical information may also be particularly relevant to primary care decision making. For example, Muris *et al.* have demonstrated that clusters of clinical information are more helpful than individual clinical characteristics in making decisions about patients with non-specific abdominal symptoms in a primary care setting (*see* Table 3.6).[16] However, careful consideration needs to be given to the potential lack of independence between items of clinical information, the net

TABLE 3.5 Variation in posterior probability according to prior probability

Prior probability, %	Prior odds	Posterior odds after applying a LR of 5	Posterior probability, %	Net increase in probability, %
10	0.11	0.55	35.5	25.5
20	0.25	1.25	55.5	35.5
30	0.43	2.15	68.3	38.3

LR = likelihood ratio

TABLE 3.6 Clinical indicants and neoplastic disease

	Probability for neoplastic disease (%)
Age > 65, male	3
Age > 65, male, non-specific abdominal pain	18
Age > 65, male, non-specific abdominal pain and weight loss	50
Age > 65, male, non-specific abdominal pain, weight loss, and ESR > 20 mm/h	75

discriminatory value of the combinations often being slightly lower than predicted from simply multiplying the likelihood ratios together.[17] For example, in relation to the diagnosis of urological cancer in patients with new-onset haematuria it seems that the unadjusted combination of male sex, hesitancy, poor stream, and having at least three episodes of haematuria overestimates the combined positive likelihood ratio by 15%.[18]

Considering decision-making thresholds and risk communication

In view of the low prevalences of many serious or important conditions within primary care, primary care physicians differ from specialists in the amount of risk they are willing to take when confronted with a particular symptom. It is invariably necessary to make a trade-off between missing cases (false negatives) and overdiagnosis (false positives). Where this point lies depends on striking a balance between the likelihood of disease in the population and the utility of making an early diagnosis and taking appropriate prompt action. If primary care clinicians adopt the same thresholds for action across the whole spectrum of disease as do their hospital colleagues they will inevitably generate much suffering through false alarms.

Over 20 years ago, Pauker and Kassirer suggested that the approach to diagnosis and treatment uses two thresholds, a 'test-no treatment' threshold and a 'test-treatment' threshold.[19]

Figure 3.4 can be used to illustrate Pauker and Kassirer's ideas modified in accordance with the primary care perspective. For example, when confronted with

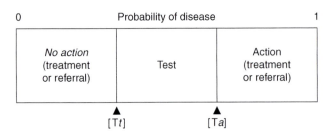

FIGURE 3.4 Decision-making thresholds

a patient complaining of tiredness, the primary care clinician may elect to take no action as they feel (perhaps based on the patient's age, sex or past history) that the probability of disease is low. In other situations the doctor may judge that the probability is a little higher and decide to subject the patient to further assessment such as taking a more detailed clinical history, performing a clinical examination or undertaking some simple investigations. Thus, in relation to the model, the physician has decided that the probability of disease has exceeded the 'test' [Tt] threshold and the process now involves the collection of additional 'test' information, until the probability of disease is either increased (to the 'action' threshold [Ta]) or reduced to below [Tt]. I have used the term 'action' rather than 'treatment' as the primary care clinician may initiate a referral in preference to treating the patient themselves.

Clearly the threshold probabilities will vary for different diseases and also depend on the discriminatory characteristics of the clinical indicants being used, the risks of the clinical indicant and the balance between the risks and the benefits of any treatment as assessed by the patient and the clinician. In some circumstances, such as the presentation of a 60-year-old man with chest pain to the primary care clinician, it is necessary to have low thresholds as patients with myocardial infarcts certainly have improved outcomes with early hospitalisation and it may even be sensible to have [Ta] very close to [Tt]. However, in contrast, referring every patient with loose motions into secondary care with a view to colonoscopy may result in significant harm. One further consideration is that as certain aspects of the clinical indicant properties give cause for concern the threshold [Ta] will approach [Tt]. In other words, if the validity or the reliability of the clinical indicant is dubious, the information may become inapplicable in relation to the amount of risk doctors are willing to accommodate.

Changes in society's expectations and increased patient autonomy are emphasising the importance of explicitly involving the patient in deciding on a particular course of action (or inaction). Communicating risk is not easy and the strength of a person's preference for a particular outcome may not match the expectations of the doctor. We also need to be aware of the multiple and conflicting sources of information to which patients have access as well as the impact of other social and psychological influences on a decision. As doctors we can also easily influence a patient's decision by how we present findings. For example, talking about the chances of survival is considerably more persuasive than focusing on the probability of death in getting an individual to select a somewhat risky option.

Supporting informed and rational decision making can involve several stages.
1   Clarifying the decision by carefully defining and explaining the problem. This should also encompass an appreciation of the uncertain nature of medical knowledge and practice.
2   Discussing the evidence base and checking patient understanding.
3   Acknowledging the patient's role in decision making.

4   Unbiased and effective communication about potential benefits and harms of different options.
5   Exploring the patient's attitudes to the benefits and harms outlined.

In communicating risks care needs to be taken with the vocabulary used as well as the denominator chosen. One person's understanding of 'likely' may be a chance of one in ten, whereas another may think it means a chance of one in two. If different denominators are used (i.e. 1/100 or 30/1000), many patients mistake which is the greater risk. Portraying options can also be difficult; for example, it is recognised that many patients find the choice 'doing nothing' unpalatable and, in this situation, the use of more positive options such as 'watchful waiting' may be more acceptable.

Once I attempted to discuss risks and benefits of colonoscopy with a fit 70-year-old woman suffering from a mild iron-deficiency anaemia. After only a few seconds, and before I had got into my stride, she interjected 'Dr Summerton, you are supposed to be the doctor and I am the patient, I want you to tell me what to do'. Clearly patients will vary in their desire to be involved in decision making as well as in their ability to assimilate and understand information and uncertainty. Primary care diagnostics is also about knowing your audience as well as the principles of risk communication, decision-making thresholds and Bayes' Theorem!

Making better use of time

Time is important to the primary care physician at a number of levels. Individual patient encounters are short, often lasting less than 10 minutes in the UK, and we need diagnostic tools that are useful and useable within this brief contact period. On the other hand, the primary care clinician frequently enjoys a long-term relationship with a patient that may influence assessment by building up a picture over several consultations and encouraging 'watchful waiting' as well as encouraging shared decision making.

It has been estimated that in the UK, the average yearly patient consultation time with their general practitioner amounts to approximately 47 minutes.[20] Knowledge gained over such a period can be particularly important in achieving a diagnosis in patients presenting with new, non-specific problems such as fever, fatigue or generalised pain to primary care physicians. Moreover, in a study of 500 adults presenting to a walk-in clinic in Washington DC with physical symptoms, 70% of patients improved within two weeks and, of the remainder, 60% were better within three months.[21]

Temporal discriminators can be of particular assistance to primary care practitioners and such discriminators may relate not only to alterations in clinical characteristics (e.g. persistence or periodicity of symptoms), but also to an individual's behaviour. Recently, when I was consulted by a gentleman with a persistent chest infection, two such temporal factors added to my concerns: he had not visited the doctor in five years and, three months before, he had suddenly stopped smoking. A subsequent chest radiograph supported the likely diagnosis of lung cancer.

Diagnosis by 'test of time' involves a careful initial assessment of the patient's presenting problem(s) followed by one or more reassessment(s) after a predefined period of time. The test of time can be particularly helpful in diagnosing patients presenting with common problems such as cough, sore throat, diarrhoea or back pain where the initial assessment has not identified any red flags and the clinical course is reasonably well established for the more common causes. However, problems can arise if the initial assessment is inadequate, if the patient fails to return for review, if the time frame for re-assessment is incorrect or if it proves too difficult to determine whether a clinically important change has occurred.

In a recent review of the 'test of time' principle, the following recommendations were made:[22]

- A careful and comprehensive initial assessment covering the presenting problem, any associated symptoms or signs, co-morbidities and the patient's current physical or emotional state should be undertaken.
- The follow-up plan should be explicit about re-assessments and must be agreed with the patient. It should be based, as far as possible, on the known course of the presenting problem and the clinically important difference than needs to be detected.
- Wherever possible, monitoring should use features that can be objectively assessed (e.g. measurement of skin lesions and lymph nodes) and that have good reliability (reproducibility).

It is also possible to make active (rather than simply passive) use of time in the context of a trial of treatment. In such circumstances the patient is given a new treatment and the subsequent clinical course can help to confirm (or exclude) a likely diagnosis. Examples include the use of corticosteroids in individuals with suspected polymyalgia rheumatica but a low or normal ESR, and trials of inhaled corticosteroids or proton pump inhibitors in individuals with chronic cough.[23,24] Unfortunately, many factors can mislead doctors (and patients) conducting such uncontrolled evaluations; these include the placebo effect, the natural history of the illness, regression to the mean, and the expectations of the patient and the clinician. Giving medications (and placebos) to patients in a randomised sequence is a more epidemiologically and statistically robust approach. In such an 'N-of-1' trial, a patient undergoes a treatment testing involving randomised pairs or triplets of treatment/placebo periods. Both the patient and the clinician are blind to allocation, and patient-oriented outcomes are carefully monitored to assess patient-specific effectiveness and the likely diagnosis.[25]

CLINICAL DECISION SUPPORT

In recent years there has been growing interest in the use of clinical decision rules (both paper-based and computerised) within primary care to enhance the accuracy of diagnostic assessments. A clinical decision rule is a clinical tool that quantifies the individual contributions that various components of the medical history, physical examination and basic investigations make towards the diagnosis, prognosis or likely response to treatment in a patient.[26]

As illustrated in Chapter 7 (deep vein thrombosis) and Chapter 8 (ankle injuries), clinical decision rules have a potential role in primary care diagnostics, but need to be carefully assessed before being used in day-to-day practice. Once a clinical decision rule has been developed it is important that its effectiveness be confirmed in patients that were not included in the development study. Subsequently work must be undertaken to determine whether its use by primary care clinicians in routine practice actually does change diagnostic and therapeutic decisions, improve patient outcomes or reduce health service costs.[27] Several features are certainly correlated with a decision support system's ability to improve the process of patient care.[28] A successful decision support system:

- is time sensitive; it permits rapid information input and produces a speedy output
- is simple to use with minimal necessary input requirements
- is integrated into the clinician's workflow and existing computer systems
- produces positive recommendations for action rather than assessments

However, according to Garg and colleagues, although many computerised clinical decision support systems certainly improve practitioner performance, the effects on patient outcomes remain understudied or inconsistent.[29] Thus, when presented with a new clinical decision rule (often by an enthusiastic hospital clinician, a commercial supplier or a health service manager) it is important to seek to classify the tool into one of four groups:

1 The rule has been evaluated in one or more routine primary care settings and has been demonstrated to change general practitioner behaviour and improve patient outcomes.
2 The rule has been evaluated in one or more routine primary care settings and has been demonstrated to change general practitioner behaviour.
3 The rule has been evaluated (although not in a routine primary care setting) and has been demonstrated to change clinician behaviour and improve patient outcomes.
4 The rule has been evaluated (although not in a routine primary care setting) and has been demonstrated to change clinician behaviour.

Ideally I should like for any diagnostic rule being promoted for use within primary care to fall into group 1.

GENERAL REFERENCES

- Armstrong BK, White E, Saracci R. *Principles of Exposure Measurement in Epidemiology*. Oxford: Oxford University Press, 1992.
- Black ER, Bordley DR, Tape TG, *et al.* editors. *Diagnostic Strategies for Common Medical Problems*. Philadelphia: American College of Physicians, 1999.
- Edwards A, Elwyn G. *Evidence-Based Patient Choice*. Oxford: Oxford University Press, 2001.
- Fletcher RH, Fletcher SW, Wagner EH. *Clinical Epidemiology: the essentials*. Baltimore: Williams & Wilkins, 1996.
- Fraser RC. *Clinical Method: a general practice approach*. Oxford: Butterworth-Heinemann, 1999.
- McWhinney IR. *A Textbook of Family Medicine*. Oxford: Oxford University Press, 1997.
- Sackett DL, Haynes RB, Guyatt GH, *et al. Clinical Epidemiology: a basic science for clinical medicine*. Boston: Little, Brown and Company, 1991.
- Streiner DL, Norman GR. *Health Measurement Scales*. Oxford: Oxford University Press, 1995.

TEXT REFERENCES

1. Howie JGR. Diagnosis – the Achilles' heel? *J Roy Coll Gen Pract* 1972; **22**: 310–15.
2. Fiscella K, Franks P, Zwanziger J, *et al.* Risk aversion and costs. A comparison of family physicians and general internists. *J Fam Pract* 2000; **49**: 12–16.
3. Hippocrates (Lloyd GER, editor). *Hippocratic Writings*. London: Penguin Books, 1978.
4. Bomback A. The physical exam and the sense of smell. *N Engl J Med* 2006; **354**: 327–9.
5. Anderson MR, Klink K, Cohrssen A. Evaluation of vaginal complaints. *JAMA* 2004; **291**: 1368–79.
6. Willis CM, Church SM, Guest CM, *et al.* Olfactory detection of bladder cancer by dogs: proof of principle study. *BMJ* 2004; **329**: 712.
7. Woodman CBJ, Richardson J, Spence M. Why do we continue to take unnecessary smears? *Brit J Gen Pract* 1997; **47**: 645–6.
8. Van Den Akker M, Buntinx F, Metsemakers JFM, *et al.* Multimorbidity in general practice: prevalence, incidence, and determinants of co-occurring chronic and recurrent diseases. *Clinical Epidemiology* 1998; **51**: 367–75.
9. Melbye H, Straume B, Brox J. Laboratory tests for pneumonia in general practice: the diagnostic values depend on the duration of illness. *Scand J Prim Health Care* 1992; **10**: 234–40.
10. Fijten GH, Starmans R, Muris JWM, *et al.* Predictive value of signs and symptoms for colorectal cancer in patients with rectal bleeding in general practice. *Family Practice* 1995; **12**: 279–86.
11. De Marco MF, Janssen-Heijnen MLG, van der Heijden LH, *et al.* Comorbidity and colorectal cancer according to subsite and stage: a population-based study. *Eur J Cancer* 2000; **36**: 95–9.

12. Hargarten SW, Roberts MJS, Anderson AJ. Cancer presentation in the emergency department: a failure of primary care. *Am J Emerg Med* 1992; **10**: 290–3.

13. Landis JR, Koch GG. The measurement of observer agreement for categorical data. *Biometrics* 1977; **33**: 671–9.

14. Sox HC, Hickman DH, Marton KI, *et al.* Using the patient's history to estimate the probability of coronary artery disease: a comparison of primary care and referral practices. *Am J Med* 1990; **89**: 7–14.

15. Okkes IM, Oskam SK, Lamberts H. The probability of specific diagnoses for patients presenting with common symptoms to Dutch family physicians. *J Fam Pract* 2002; **51**: 31–6.

16. Muris JWM, Starmans R, Fijten GH, *et al.* Non-acute abdominal complaints in general practice: diagnostic value of signs and symptoms. *Brit J Gen Pract* 1995; **45**: 313–16.

17. Summerton N. The medical history as a diagnostic technology. *Brit J Gen Pract* 2008; **58**: 273–6.

18. Summerton N, Mann S, Rigby AS, *et al.* Patients with new onset haematuria: assessing the discriminant value of clinical information in relation to urological malignancies. *Brit J Gen Pract* 2002; **52**: 284–9.

19. Pauker SG, Kassirer JP. The threshold approach to clinical decision making. *N Engl J Med* 1980; **302**: 1109–17.

20. Pereira-Gray DJ. Forty-seven minutes for the patient. *Brit J Gen Pract* 1998; **48**: 1816–17.

21. Kroenke K, Jackson JL. Outcome in general medical patients presenting with common symptoms: a prospective study with a 2-week and a 3-month follow-up. *Family Practice* 1998; **15**: 398–403.

22. Almond SC, Summerton N. Diagnosis in general practice: Test of time. *BMJ* 2009; **338**: 1878–80.

23. Glasziou P, Rose P, Heneghan C, Balla J. Diagnosis in general practice: Diagnosis using "test of treatment". *BMJ* 2009; **338**: 1267–9.

24. Barraclough K. Diagnosis in general practice: Chronic cough in adults. *BMJ* 2009; **338**: 1267–9.

25. Summerton N. Optimising treatments in primary care using single patient tests. *Future Prescriber* 2003; **4**: 22–4.

26. McGinn TG, Guyatt GH, Wyer PC, *et al.* Users' guides to the medical literature XXII: How to use articles about clinical decision rules. *JAMA* 2000; **284**: 79–84.

27. Toll DB, Janssen KJM, Vergouwe Y, Moons KGM. Validation, updating and impact of clinical prediction rules: a review. *J Clin Epidemiol* 2008; **61**: 1085–94.

28. Kawamoto K, Houlihan CA, Balas EA, Lobach DF. Improving clinical practice using clinical decision support systems: a systematic review of trials to identify features critical to success. *BMJ* 2005; **330**: 765–8.

29. Garg AX, Adhikari NKJ, McDonald H, *et al.* Effects of computerised clinical decision support systems on practitioner performance and patient outcomes. *JAMA* 2005; **293**: 1223–38.

CHAPTER 4

Patient's story: symptoms

INTRODUCTION

In Chapter 2 the general importance of the medical history in achieving diagnoses and making rational patient-centred decisions were highlighted. However, taking a medical history is not merely about the assembly of facts concerning a patient's presenting problem, their previous healthcare history, medication use, family history, health behaviours, occupational history or social history, it also involves the careful interpretation and appraisal of the information obtained. This chapter focuses on symptoms and in Chapter 5 I look at some aspects of the previous healthcare history, health behaviour and the family history.

SYMPTOMS

Symptoms have a long pedigree. Hippocrates recognised their key role in patient care and the term 'symptom' comes from the Greek *symptoma* which means 'anything that has befallen one'; the Greek verb is *piptein* 'to fall'.[1] Thus a symptom is a fall from the usual state of functioning. I find writing difficult; it is even harder when I am tired and have a headache!

Symptoms are the commonest reason for a patient to consult a doctor and yet their diagnostic importance has been incrementally downgraded over the last century. For example, as a general practitioner, I often measure FSH (follicle-stimulating hormone) levels in women who I suspect may be perimenopausal. But, according to a review, the best predictors that a woman will enter menopause within four years are: age at least 50 years, amenorrhoea for 3 to 11 months and menstrual cycle irregularity within 12 months.[2] Until recently I continued to argue that the clinical question of perimenopausal status was more challenging for patients in their early to mid-40s and, in this group, it was still reasonable to check FSH levels to confirm the diagnosis. However, I was eventually forced to change my view by Bastian *et al.* who collated information on positive likelihood ratios in addition to negative likelihood ratios.[3] The results are given in Table 4.1.

These figures indicate that, even on their own, hot flushes are a better discriminator than FSH measurement. Moreover, taken together with night sweats, vaginal

TABLE 4.1 Clinical information and menopausal status

Clinical information	Positive likelihood ratio	Negative likelihood ratio
Hot flushes	3.2	0.7
Night sweats	1.9	0.8
Vaginal dryness	2.6	0.9
Patient's self-rating of going through the transition	1.8	0.3
FSH (>24 IU/L)	3.1	0.5

dryness and self-rating, the total positive likelihood ratio could possibly be as high as 28.5. Conversely, to rule out perimenopause, the patient's self-rating had a negative likelihood ratio closer to zero than did FSH measurement.

Urinary tract infections are another common problem in general practice and many of us will base our prescribing decisions on the identification of abnormalities on dipstick or culture rather than the patient's symptoms. Interestingly, a recent randomised controlled trial demonstrated that in women with dysuria and frequency but a negative urine dipstick result for nitrates and leucocytes, three out of four will respond to antibiotics compared with one out of four taking placebo.[4]

The patient-symptom dyad lies at the heart of primary care diagnostics. Unexplored, unexplained and unresolved symptoms can lead to patient dissatisfaction and longer term morbidity. Moreover, unnecessary or unwarranted investigation of inadequately explored symptoms can result in considerable physical and psychological harm, irrespective of the wastage of scarce healthcare resources.

It is also important to appreciate that in some situations the absence of specific symptoms may have greater diagnostic value than their presence. In patients with lung disease, the presence of orthopnoea has limited value as it occurs in both lung and heart disease. However the *absence* of orthopnoea strongly argues against the presence of associated left ventricular dysfunction (negative likelihood ratio = 0.04).[5]

PATIENT-CENTRED INTERVIEWING

Patient-centred interviewing is about actively listening and clarifying the patient's story and symptom history as well as extracting additional items of clinical information during the course of a conversation. Some would argue that this can be equally effectively achieved by interrogating a patient using a questionnaire or a computer and there is certainly evidence that the information gained using these mechanisms can be as good as that obtained by a doctor. However, the question needs to be considered as to whether such equivalence really reflects inadequacies in the doctor's interviewing skills rather than the technical wizardry of the computer. Responding to verbal and non-verbal clues given out by patients certainly requires human interaction.

I can well remember a 19-year-old girl with mild (and well-controlled) schizophrenia who came to see me at the start of a university term complaining of 'feeling cold'. I took a cursory history, undertook a somewhat perfunctory examination and arranged a number of simple investigations all of which turned out to be normal. Adopting a rather 'doctor-centred' style, I put the symptom down to her medication and arranged to review the patient a few weeks later in November. When she returned she looked very smart and well but complained that the symptom of 'coldness' was considerably worse. Thankfully the reception staff had asked me to check on her current address as, if I had not, I may never have discovered that she had been forced to leave home and was sleeping rough. Once she had been found some new accommodation her symptom of 'extreme coldness' resolved.

An effective patient-centred diagnostic consultation can be characterised by a number of key tasks.
1   Making the patient feel valued and recognised as an individual.
2   Clarifying the reason(s) for the consultation.
3   Considering the relevance of any on-going problems, contextual issues and risk factors.
4   Achieving a shared understanding of the problem with the patient.
5   Agreeing the next steps with the patient.

The key to patient-centred interviewing is to allow as much as possible to flow from the patient. Primary care diagnostics is also about not dismissing or ignoring symptoms that do not make sense from the doctor's perspective. Evidence continues to accumulate about symptoms; for example, despite what I have said to patients over the years about headaches and mild hypertension, it now seems that I may have been wrong. A systematic review concluded that commonly used antihypertensive drugs reduce the prevalence of headaches by one-third compared with placebo.[6] A complex or confusing symptom presentation can be helpful in pointing us towards a psychological problem. There might also be some truth in the aphorism 'patients who make me feel anxious have anxiety, patients who make me feel depressed are depressed and patients who make me feel confused are psychotic'.

As a busy general practitioner one of the worries I have always had about patient-centred interviewing is that I might lose control of the consultation and my surgeries could end up overrunning. I know that I certainly have a tendency to interrupt patients' opening statements, and research amongst a large group of doctors has demonstrated that, on average, such interruptions occur after only 18 seconds. However, (and reassuringly for me!) it seems that when patients are uninterrupted their opening statements only last, on average, two and a half minutes. Such patients are also more likely to state their main complaint and express their real concerns.

Allowing the patient to make an opening statement without interruption also minimises the risk that 'hidden agendas' will be revealed later on in the consultation. But it is always important to tailor the approach to the individual: when I kept silent recently a rather exasperated patient eventually said 'come on doctor, ask me some questions'!

In the era of 'paper-less' practices one of my greatest difficulties is to hear, remember and to interpret the verbal and non-verbal communications revealed during the course of the opening statement. As I have not yet managed to master 'touch typing', I still smuggle a piece of paper into the consultation. This allows me the opportunity to jot down key information without looking away from the patient or accompanying them with my tuneless keyboard tapping.

Once the patient has completed their opening statement we then need to explore the issues raised and check back with the patient that our understanding and interpretation is correct. Questions are generally classified as either 'open-ended' or 'closed-ended'. Open-ended questions are those to which no answers are offered by the doctor. Closed-ended questions are questions for which a range of possible answers is specified by the clinician and the patient is simply required to make a choice from amongst the answers provided. In general, considerably more useful diagnostic information is obtained by open-ended questioning.

The following additional issues also need to be borne in mind when interrogating patients.

- Will the words be understood by the patient?
- Does the question contain abbreviations, unconventional phrases or jargon?
- Is it vague?
- Is it too precise?
- Is it biased?
- Is it threatening?
- Does it contain more than one concept?
- Does it contain a double negative?
- Are the answers mutually exclusive?
- Does it assume too much about the patient's behaviour?
- Is an unambiguous time reference provided?
- Is the question cryptic?

Probes are additional questions asked or statements made by the interviewer when the answer given by the patient is incomplete or irrelevant. In relation to the use of symptoms for diagnostic purposes it is particularly important to probe 'don't know' responses. Such probing may involve simply repeating the question, silence (the 'expectant pause') or repeating the reply, which might encourage the patient to be more forthcoming. Neutral questions or comments may also help to clarify issues (e.g. 'what do you mean by…?'), to enhance specificity (e.g. 'can you be more exact?'), and for completeness (e.g. 'anything else?').

Patient-centred interviewing is really just one element of the patient-centred clinical method advocated by Stewart *et al.* The key components are detailed in Box 4.1 and interested readers are referred to the general references at the end of this chapter for more information on this approach and the other consultation models developed by Bryne and Long, Stott and Davis, Pendleton and Neighbour.

Box 4.1 The six components of the patient-centred clinical method

1 Exploring and interpreting both the disease and the patient's illness experience (feelings, ideas, functions and expectations).
2 Understanding the whole person (i.e. the patient's unique personality, life story, and the context [environment] in which they live).
3 Finding common ground with the patient about the problem and its management. This involves defining the problem, establishing the goal of management and identifying the roles to be assumed by the doctor and the patient.
4 Incorporating prevention and health promotion.
5 Enhancing the doctor–patient relationship.
6 Being realistic about time and resources.

Primary care diagnostics must be oriented towards patient-centred outcomes. If the initial interview produces a common and shared understanding of the symptom(s) then it is likely that any therapeutic interventions (even if only simple reassurance) will be considerably more effective. For example, in a study of the headache, the most important factor predicting recovery was that the patients concerned had had a good opportunity to discuss their problems with the doctor.[7] Amongst patients presenting to their doctor with new symptoms, the factor most strongly associated with recovery at 1 month was the patient's complete agreement with the doctor's opinion.

Unfortunately, although patient-centred interviewing is an essential component of primary care diagnosis, it is not sufficient on its own. For doctors seeking to practise primary care diagnostics there is a further requirement to make judgements about the reliability and the validity of the symptom-related information offered by the patient as well as any additional information obtained by the doctor. It is particularly important not only to be aware of the value but also the limitations of a patient's description of their symptoms.

In order to facilitate this process there is a need to define, classify and categorise symptoms in addition to considering the symptom in context.

DEFINING SYMPTOMS

One of the greatest difficulties encountered in seeking to use symptoms as a diagnostic tool is the imprecise nature of symptom definitions by doctors. In some

TABLE 4.2 Suggested definitions for selected gastrointestinal symptoms

Symptom	Definition
Epigastric bloating	Sensation of abdominal distension
Early satiety	Not being able to complete a normal-sized meal
Postprandial nausea	Sick feeling after a meal
Vomiting	Bringing up of food or fluid preceded or accompanied by a sick feeling
Regurgitation	Bringing up of fluid not preceded or accompanied by a sick feeling
Heartburn	Burning sensation behind the sternum, aggravated by lying down, stooping, large meals

early work on dyspepsia, De Dombal found this issue particularly perplexing, as it seemed that doctors' ideas about the meaning of key symptoms were amazingly variable.[8] The understanding of terms such as 'early satiety', 'heartburn', 'regurgitation' and even 'vomiting' varied between doctors. This situation is analogous to scientists having a range of definitions for basic physical terms such as mass, density or force! A diagnostic pathway that commences with an ill-defined symptom is therefore fundamentally flawed and, more worryingly, subsequent steps in the diagnostic processing will simply perpetuate and even magnify this initial error.

In my view, symptoms are only useful for diagnostic purposes (both for clinical practice and for clinical research) if they can be consistently defined and if these definitions are agreed between doctors and learnt by medical students. As a starting point De Dombal suggested the definitions shown in Table 4.2 for a number of gastrointestinal-related symptoms.[8]

CLASSIFYING SYMPTOMS

Once a symptom has been defined, it then needs to be categorised. I find the following symptom classification helpful in practising primary care diagnostics as it assists me in being clearer about the broad type of symptom that I am facing.

'Normal' symptoms

Frequently we encounter patients with a symptom that may be quite 'normal' for them. Some patients become concerned if they do not have a daily bowel action and others seem to be particularly troubled by physiological vaginal discharge. It is important to be aware of such normal symptoms as excessive investigation of them can easily lead to unnecessary distress for patients. For example, it appears that a normal vaginal discharge increases at mid-cycle, can be malodorous, and may even be accompanied by irritative symptoms such as itch.[9]

It would also seem reasonable to suggest that, for some symptoms, there is a normal distribution or variation for the symptom and the issue is to decide at what point it should be classified as 'abnormal' and further investigations initiated. We all get an occasional headache, experience pain or feel tired. However, if the headache persists, becomes more severe or frequent we might consider it 'abnormal'. Primary care diagnostics is about involving the patient in setting the threshold for normality. One approach is to use quantifying questions such as the following.

- Has the dizziness been a *major* problem for you?
- Have you been bothered *a lot* by headaches?
- Have you had trouble with *excessive* wind?

Iatrotropic symptoms

Iatrotropic symptoms (from the Greek *iatros* [doctor] and *trope* [turn]) are those symptoms that lead a patient to seek medical advice from a doctor.[10] They need to be distinguished from the non-iatrotropic symptoms that are only disclosed during the course of the clinical interview. Obviously a symptom can fall into either group but some are clearly more likely to be iatrotropic than others.

Especially where the iatrotropic symptom is vague or of little interest to me, I often find my questioning drifting towards the more 'doctor-centred', non-iatrotropic symptoms. It takes considerable discipline to re-focus on the patient's concerns and it is an interesting exercise in primary care diagnostics to ask patients to jot down their major problem(s) while they are sitting in the waiting room.

Unfortunately many patients may not appreciate which symptoms matter in terms of, for example, earlier cancer diagnosis and therefore warrant a consultation. Walker demonstrated that only 50% of women were aware that post-menopausal bleeding could be a symptom of cancer and only 57% of women realised that a painless breast lump could be malignant.[11] In a Dutch study, Huygen found that 12% of the 631 respondents to a survey were experiencing potentially serious symptoms but did not consider consulting a doctor.[12] Primary care diagnostics is therefore also about marrying up the patient's expertise about their symptom with the doctor's expertise about the likely diagnostic significance of that symptom in relation to serious and important conditions.

To complicate matters further a patient's presenting symptom may be merely a 'ticket for admission' in order to focus on other concerns. It can take some skill in patient-centred interviewing to get beneath the pseudo-iatrotropic symptom in order to reach the true iatrotropic symptom. I can recall a patient who came to see me with a testicular swelling who confessed that he had recently been to see another primary care physician but, having felt unable to mention his testicular problem to a female doctor, stated that he had a sore throat and earache. Aside from his testicular swelling he was now also uncertain as to whether he should complete his course of antibiotics and attend the ear, nose and throat outpatient appointment arranged for him!

It is important to appreciate that personal, psychological, social and economic factors can all lower the threshold for iatrotropy. However, in general, certain symptoms are more likely to lead to a doctor consultation than others (*see* Table 4.3).[13]

TABLE 4.3 Symptoms and consultations amongst younger women

Symptom	Ratio of symptom episodes to consultation
Changes in energy	456:1
Headache	184:1
Disturbance of gastric function	109:1
Backache	52:1
Pain in lower limb	49:1
Abdominal pain	29:1
Sore throat	18:1
Pain in chest	14:1

In the previous chapter I discussed Bayes' Theorem and its application to diagnostic decision making. The calculation is achieved using odds, i.e.:

posterior odds = likelihood ratio × prior odds*

However, the sequence is most easily understood in terms of probabilities.*

Patient presentation (e.g. with symptom) (prior probability)

Likelihood ratios from history

Post-history probability

Likelihood ratios from examination

Post-examination probability

Likelihood ratios from testing

Post-test probability (posterior probability)

The group of patients presenting with an iatrotropic symptom such as haematuria who subsequently turn out to have a urological malignancy represents the prior odds (or prior probability). Non-iatrotropic information (i.e. information obtained during

---

*See Glossary.

the course of the interview about other symptoms (e.g. hesitancy of micturition) in addition to more detailed information about the iatrotropic symptom (e.g. number of episodes of haematuria) can be assigned likelihood ratios which will act to adjust the post-history probability of disease. In our own study of haematuria the prior probability could be increased from 9.9% (based on the iatrotropic group) to a post-history probability of 69% after the application of a number of positive likelihood ratios (e.g. hesitancy of micturition gave a positive likelihood ratio of 5.9 and three instances of haematuria rather than one gave a positive likelihood ratio of 2.7).[14]

In seeking to undertake clinically relevant diagnostic research it is important to differentiate between those symptoms that cause a patient to consult and those which we might subsequently wish to enquire about in the context of this symptom-defined grouping (*see also* Chapter 8). Simply grouping together symptoms irrespective of which symptom brought the patient to the doctor may count as diagnostic research but it is of doubtful relevance to the types of patient encountered on a day-to-basis in primary care.

Objective/non-sensory symptoms

Personally I know that I am much more comfortable with objective symptoms such as haemoptysis or haematuria than I am with the more subjective symptoms of dizziness, tiredness, abdominal pain or headache. I find that dizziness is more difficult and time consuming to unravel, whereas symptoms such as weight loss or bleeding can be independently verified and measured. There is often a temptation to go for the (often secondary) objective and non-sensory symptoms or to simply reach for the pathology request form!

Unfortunately subjective symptoms are common and in a community survey of symptoms the most prevalent symptoms reported are listed in Table 4.4.[15]

TABLE 4.4 Subjective symptoms in the community

Symptom	Prevalence (%)
Joint pain	36.7
Back pain	31.5
Headache	24.9
Chest pain	24.6
Arm or leg pain	24.3
Abdominal pain	23.6
Fatigue	23.6
Dizziness	23.2
Insomnia	19.2
Dysuria	19.2
Trouble walking	18.3
Palpitations	18.2

The preference for objective symptoms by many doctors may reflect something about our training in terms of both the emphasis on scientific measurement and the differences in the balance of sensory and non-sensory symptoms between secondary care and primary care.

However, from the patient's perspective, it seems that the subjective sensations are often the most perplexing. Primary care diagnostics must therefore be about clinicians and clinical researchers actually concentrating on those problems that concern patients. Inadequately explored subjective symptoms inevitably end up requiring more investigation in the longer term that is considerably more expensive. In such circumstances a poor initial interview represents a significant opportunity cost.

Somatic symptoms

One particular problem for those of us working in primary care settings (i.e. the first port of call for patients) is that the vast majority of symptoms we encounter seem to defy a clear-cut organic explanation. Kroenke and Mangelsdorff demonstrated that no specific physical disorder could be established as the cause in 30–75% of instances, even after careful investigation.[16] Table 4.5 shows the proportions of six common symptoms with likely organic aetiologies presenting to US primary care physicians over a 3-year period.

Furthermore, in relation to specific symptoms such as chest pain, it seems that primary care physicians are more likely to encounter patients with psychological causes than with serious lung or cardiovascular conditions in comparison with hospital-based clinical colleagues.[17]

Somatic symptoms (or functional symptoms) are defined as symptoms (objective or subjective; iatrotropic or non-iatrotropic) without an organic cause. However, it is very important to appreciate that such 'medically unexplained symptoms' are not synonymous with 'unimportant symptoms'.

Depression and anxiety often present with somatic symptoms that can resolve with effective treatment of these disorders. In fact it is suggested that the vast majority

TABLE 4.5 Proportions of six common symptoms with a suspected organic cause

Symptom	Probable organic aetiology (%)
Chest pain	11
Fatigue	13
Dizziness	18
Headache	10
Back pain	10
Abdominal pain	10

of patients with depression in primary care present with physical, not emotional, complaints.[18] Classical somatic symptoms in depressed individuals are headache, constipation, weakness, fatigue, abdominal pain, insomnia, anorexia and weight loss. Anxiety-related manifestations include headache, gastrointestinal disturbances such as diarrhoea and cramps, musculoskeletal pain, palpitations, dyspnoea, sweating and fainting.

Antidepressants can be highly effective in depressed patients presenting with somatic symptoms. There is also good evidence that antidepressants often help even when there are no clear symptoms of depression. Furthermore, patients with identifiable organic causes for their symptoms may also have functional elements.[19] Somatic symptoms resulting from anxiety and depression are common in patients with cardiovascular diseases and untreated psychiatric disorders in these patients worsens prognosis.

Obviously, it is always necessary to exclude organic disease when presented with a symptom of possible organic significance such as unexplained weight loss, chest pain or palpitations. However, I am confident that, as a primary care clinician, I am not unique in falling into the trap of undertaking investigations beyond those that are absolutely necessary. For example, Kroenke argues that abdominal pain and chest pain considered non-organic after the initial primary care assessment are seldom harbingers of serious disorder during long-term follow-up.[20] Muris *et al.* discovered that, of those who initially had unexplained abdominal symptoms, 68% experienced complete relief or improvement after one year and that depressive mood was associated with the persistence of symptoms.[21]

An organically-oriented mindset can also lead to beliefs in spurious associations or pseudo-relationships between symptoms and diseases. In a study of general surgical patients, it was found that so called 'biliary pain' was not consistently related to gall-stone disease, although this is often the only feature that was used to determine the requirement for surgical intervention.[22] I know that I am more likely to order blood counts in patients complaining of fatigue than amongst those who do not. Consequently, within the group of patients I subsequently diagnose as having anaemia there will be a greater proportion complaining of fatigue than within the unselected general practice population. Although well-conducted population studies have demonstrated no link between fatigue and anaemia, my personal experience continues to mislead me.

In our society there is a stigma associated with psychological illness compounded by a perception that all symptoms need to be explained in mechanistic (and even molecular) terms. This impacts on all of us and it is all-to-easy to over-investigate such patients in order to avoid leaving any 'organic' stone unturned. According to McWhinney, the doctor-centred model of clinical decision making places a high value on seeking greater precision. Unfortunately this does not necessarily reduce uncertainty or lead to a more accurate definition of the problem. There is a further issue: patients themselves may have recognised that there is a psychological dimension to their symptom and become sceptical about our ability to help them with this.

I find the following list helpful in reminding me to consider the possibility of a somatic symptom.

1 Frequent attendance with the same symptoms.
2 Large numbers of symptoms.
3 Attendances with a symptom that has been present for a long time.
4 Incongruity between the patient's distress and the comparatively minor nature of the symptoms.
5 Inability to make sense of the presenting problem.

Nowadays if I think a symptom is likely to be somatic (or functional) I have learnt to state my position in the initial conversation with the patient. During the course of undertaking any necessary investigations, a further explanation about the causes of symptoms is then provided and is discussed. Throughout the initial and subsequent encounters I believe primary care diagnostics must also incorporate a shared understanding of the benefits of increasing diagnostic precision weighed against the hazards of further investigation. In The Netherlands primary care physicians are discouraged from rushing to investigate complaints unexplained after taking an adequate history and conducting a competent clinical examination for a least four weeks after first presentation as the probability that such a patient will be suffering from an, as yet, undetectable disease is very low.

Indirect symptoms

In the sub-section on iatrotropic symptoms I introduced the concept of pseudo-iatrotropic symptoms to indicate that some symptoms may simply serve as an excuse to see a doctor. There is also some evidence that entry into consultation can be by means of symptoms in a friend or relative. For example, childhood consultations may sometimes be more about the mother's symptoms and concerns that those of the child. Occasionally when two or three individuals come into my consulting room there may be some confusion as to who is actually presenting with the clinical problem! Despite the most tightly designed appointments systems and restrictions on furniture, patients who have the appointment still often ask me to just 'check over' their friend, relative or child.

CATEGORISATION OF SYMPTOMS

Once a symptom has been identified the next step is to explore the details of that symptom. Temporal variability, quantity and quality, location, aggravating and alleviating factors and associated features may all provide diagnostic clues. However, in making sense of these symptom categorisations it is also helpful to use operational definitions for imprecise terms. For example, shortness of breath might be subdivided into mild dyspnoea if it does not limit normal activity, moderate dyspnoea if it limits but does not prevent normal activity and severe dyspnoea if it prevents normal activity.

In seeking to practise primary care diagnostics there is also a need to be confident about the validity of the symptom categorisations being used. These should be based on the best available evidence derived from research conducted amongst the groups of patients we are likely to encounter in day-to-day primary care clinical practice. For example, Thiadens *et al.* discovered that in patients with persistent cough presenting to general practitioners a scoring system based on one detailed feature of the iatrotropic symptom (aggravation by fog, smoke, exercise or cold air) and two associated symptoms (wheeze and dyspnoea) correctly identified most patients with COPD or asthma.[23]

Palpitations represent one of the most common symptoms in general medical settings, reported by as many as 16% of patients. In most cases palpitations are not associated with structural heart disease. They may be provoked by a host of factors including exercise, emotional stress and fever. In our own work studying patients presenting to a group of 62 general practitioners with new-onset palpitations, symptom-related information obtained from these patients was compared against the results from a *RhythmCard* event recorder (the reference standard). We discovered that those with regular palpitations and those experiencing palpitations at work were significantly more likely to have a cardiac cause for their palpitations. There also appeared to be a dose–response effect with duration; the longer the palpitation lasted the more likely that it represented a significant cardiac arrhythmia.[24]

SYMPTOMS IN CONTEXT

As mentioned earlier in this chapter, the key to patient-centred interviewing is to allow as much as possible to flow from the patient. This is not only about symptoms but also information about expectations, thoughts, feelings and fears. Symptoms can only really be interpreted in context and it has even been suggested that doctors should base their diagnoses on symptom presentations rather than specific symptoms.

Primary care diagnostics is about focusing on the interaction between the patient and the physician in the context of primary care. However, aside from this, there are at least three other dimensions that need to be considered when interpreting a symptom: patient, time and environment.

The patient dimension
Demographics
Age, sex, ethnicity and socioeconomic state can all impact on the community prevalence of symptoms as well as the iatrotropic thresholds for particular symptoms and symptom groups. In one study, 56% of Asian adults with headache consulted their

general practitioner compared with 24% for non-Asians. For tiredness, the respective figures were 33% and 12%.[25]

During an acute myocardial infarction women are more likely than men to report shortness of breath, nausea, vomiting, back pain, jaw pain, neck pain, cough and fatigue but less likely than men to report chest pain and sweating.[26] In relation to melanomas older patients more commonly report ulceration than do younger patients.[27] The threshold for doctor consultation with children is also generally lower than in adults.

Co-morbidity

In persons over the age of 65, nearly one-quarter will be suffering from one or more chronic diseases. Such co-existing problems (and their treatments) can impact on symptom presentations. For example, patients with coronary heart disease who also have diabetes are more likely to present with dyspnoea than individuals without diabetes. Conversely, symptoms thought to be diagnostic of ischaemic heart disease might not be helpful in patients with diabetes.[28] Autonomic neuropathy may predispose to infarction and result in atypical presenting symptoms in the diabetic patient. Patients with diabetes are also more likely to experience upper and lower gastrointestinal symptoms even after taking into account any side-effects of treatments that they may be receiving.[29] In patients with chronic renal disease, dyspnoea, weight loss and chest pain were shown to be the most common presenting symptoms for lung cancer diagnosis in one series.[30]

Communication and language

One of the greatest difficulties in using symptoms as diagnostic tools is the communication gap between doctors and patients. When a patient states that they are 'dizzy' it is important to establish precisely what he or she means by dizziness. Vertigo is when patients have a sensation of movement (often horizontal or rotatory) either of themselves or their surroundings and is generally due to vestibular disorders. However, 'dizziness' may also be due to psychiatric conditions, cerebrovascular disease or cardiac arrhythmias. In a group of older patients the causes shown in Table 4.6 were identified.[31]

If a patient states that they have 'spat up some blood' (an objective symptom) it is necessary to determine if they are referring to haemoptysis or haematemesis. According to Sapira a good rule of thumb is to require that the patient has actually gagged and regurgitated the bolus of blood for it to qualify as haematemesis.[32] On the other hand a patient with haemoptysis can generally recall a clear episode of coughing, but distinguishing a thoracic from a sinus origin can still be quite tricky.

Even if doctors correctly and consistently define the patient's iatrotropic symptom there is still no guarantee that the patient is using the same language or understands technical medical terms and questions. Boyle evaluated variations in the

TABLE 4.6 Cause of dizziness in 149 elderly subjects of mean age 76 years

Diagnosis	Number of subjects
Cerebrovascular disease	105
Cervical spondylosis	98
Anxiety or hyperventilation	48
Poor vision	23
Postural hypotension	14
Benign positional vertigo	6
Other	38
No diagnosis	6
More than one diagnosis	126

meanings of some commonly used medical terms utilising short multiple-choice questionnaires completed by doctors and patients.[33] The differences in the understanding of diarrhoea, flatulence and palpitations are shown in Table 4.7.

TABLE 4.7 Definitions of diarrhoea, flatulence and palpitations

Definition	Patient (%)	Doctor (%)
Diarrhoea:		
passing loose bowel motions	37.0	68.6
opening one's bowels more than once a day	3.7	nil
passing a lot of bowel motions in a short time	54.6	31.4
straining to pass bowel motions	3.7	nil
passing a lot of wind by the back passage	0.9	nil
Flatulence:		
passage of wind through the mouth or back passage	42.9	100
passage of loose bowel movements	1.9	nil
a sort of chest pain	9.5	nil
an acid taste in the mouth – especially after eating food	29.5	nil
stomach ache – usually after eating food	0.9	nil
Palpitations:		
a feeling of breathlessness – especially when excited	26.2	nil
a feeling of fright and panic	14.6	nil
a dull ache over the heart	nil	nil
a pain in the chest, usually over the heart	6.8	nil
a feeling of the heart thumping inside the chest	52.4	100

TABLE 4.8 Variation in positive responses between doctors

Symptom	Interviewer A positive response (%)	Interviewer B positive response (%)	Interviewer C positive response (%)	Interviewer D positive response (%)
Cough	23	28	40	33
Sputum	13	20	36	42
Tightness of chest	15	1	23	2
Pain	7	6	9	17
Dyspnoea	16	18	14	10

Misunderstandings can apply to adverbs and adjectives in addition to nouns and verbs. Even if doctors can agree about the terms 'productive' cough, 'rapid' breathing or 'bright-red' bleeding, there is no certainty that patients will share our understanding. The meanings of the words 'often', 'seldom' and 'rarely' can be particularly difficult to pin down.

If a large enough sample of patients is randomly divided into groups then it might be expected that the proportions reporting specific symptoms to doctors in each group would be very similar. However, in questioning a group of English coal miners about five symptoms (cough, sputum, tightness of chest, pain and dyspnoea) there were significant differences between the responses to different interviewers as shown in Table 4.8.[34]

Doctors may vary in their ability to elicit information about symptoms from patients by virtue of, perhaps, differences in the way questions are asked or the means by which any responses are explored. It also seems that personality, sex, race and age of the interviewer can also impact on the patient's responses.

To avoid problems in relation to the diagnostic use of non-iatrotropic symptoms, doctors must be careful to frame questions according to the patient's intellectual and educational level. There is also a requirement to ask questions, to clarify comprehension and to interpret responses consistently. Nobody wants to appear foolish and it is all-to-easy for patients to say 'yes or no' rather than to indicate poor understanding of the doctor. It also seems that the sequencing of questions can alter a patient's response and it is often helpful to ask the same question in different ways and at different points during the course of the history and the examination.

Cognitive state

Patients' memories can be very unreliable both due to loss of relevant information (fog) as well as the fabrication of misinformation (mirages). For example, when a group of primary care patients underwent an identical interview 1 year apart, 43% of the symptoms reported initially were not recalled 12 months later.

TABLE 4.9 Symptom agreements

Symptom	Kappa	Level of agreement
Constant cough	0.76	Substantial
Indigestion/heartburn	0.77	Substantial
Abdominal pain or discomfort	0.69	Substantial
Vomited blood during last 6 months	0.75	Substantial
Coughed up blood during last 6 months	0.73	Substantial
Blood in motions/toilet pan or on toilet paper during last 6 months	0.85	Almost perfect
Change in number of bowel movements during last 6 months	0.79	Substantial
Change in consistency of bowel movements during last 6 months	0.80	Substantial
Involuntary weight loss within last 6 months	0.84	Substantial

Various co-morbidities such as diabetes and vascular disease can also affect an individual's memory.

In general, the seriousness of a symptom or symptom-related episode and its novelty or uniqueness makes it more likely that it is recalled reliably and consistently. Also it seems that events (e.g. rectal bleeding) are remembered better than intensities (i.e. the amount of rectal bleeding). Unfortunately some patients can be coaxed into remembering symptoms that never occurred.

In my own practice patients were questioned 1 month apart about ten symptoms of possible oncological significance.[35] In order to assess the chance-corrected proportional agreement for the repeat questioning, weighted kappa was used (*see* Table 4.9). As has already been mentioned in Chapter 3, kappa values greater than 0.80 may be taken to represent almost perfect agreement, values between 0.61 and 0.80 substantial agreement, values between 0.41 and 0.60 moderate agreement, values between 0.21 and 0.40 slight agreement and values of 0.20 or below poor agreement beyond chance.

As Table 4.9 shows, for the majority of symptom reports there was substantial agreement between the two interviews. However, some symptoms are clearly more reliable than others: the question on blood in the motions/toilet pan or on the toilet paper demonstrated almost perfect agreement.

Memory for dates is particularly troublesome and the longer ago a symptom occurred the more unreliable will be the recall. In one study some patients misdated an event that had occurred within the past 4 months by as much as 3 months. Symptoms occurring a long time ago are also often displaced forward in time and recalled as having affected the patient more recently, a phenomenon referred to as 'forward telescoping'. Further confusion might arise as a number or a series of symptoms that are similar in nature may be 're-composed' as a single event.

TABLE 4.10 Change in bowel habit – agreement between questions

Symptom	Kappa	Level of agreement
Change in the number of bowel movements over a 6-month period	0.55	Moderate
Change in the consistency of bowel movements over a 6-month period	0.51	Moderate

In our own work we examined the meaning of the term 'change in bowel habit' which is traditionally taught as a feature of colorectal cancer. At one level we simply asked patients the following.

- 'Over the last 6 months have you noticed any change in the weekly number of bowel movements/motions?'
- 'Over the last 6 months have you noticed any change in the consistency of your bowel movements/motions?'

Four more detailed questions then enquired separately about the form and the frequency of the bowel movements/motions now and at a point 6 months previously by asking patients to select one of five possible categories in response to each question. The agreement in the results obtained from these two distinct approaches to questioning are shown in Table 4.10.

Thus, although a change in consistency or number of bowel movements over a 6-month period showed substantial agreement in response to the simple questions, when patients were asked more specific questions on these features currently as well as 6 months previously, the agreement was only moderate.

Corroboration (e.g. from friends and relatives) and symptom diaries are also helpful mechanisms to improve the reliability of symptom reporting. However, it is important to be aware that to keep a diary requires time and motivation and not all patients will have the necessary skills in measurement and recording. Furthermore, the act of keeping the diary may in itself affect the information being recorded.

Current health state and health beliefs

A patient's current health state and health beliefs can influence their recall of symptoms. A patient experiencing anxiety and/or depression is more likely to remember negative or unpleasant symptoms. A similar effect is noted for physical health with current pain prompting the recall of similar pain that did not come to mind when the person was pain free. Patients with chronic headache report past headaches as more intense when they were actually experiencing a headache as opposed to when they were asymptomatic. If women are asked to rate their usual degree of menstrual distress while they were menstruating they reported systematically higher levels than if they are asked the same question during the inter-menstrual phase.

Health beliefs can also impact on symptom reporting, as once a patient is labelled as 'sick' there is a tendency to underestimate symptoms in the period before they felt they became ill. This phenomenon has certainly been noted amongst patients with whiplash injury. Intriguingly, it also seems that informing healthy volunteers that they have just tested positive for a disease causes them to recall previously unreported symptoms that they had previously been told characterised that disease.

In order to take account of some of these patient dimensions in interpreting symptoms, Barsky has made the following suggestions.

- Note and take into account the patient's current physical and emotional state.
- Establish historical 'anchor points' or memorable personal or cultural milestones (such as beginning a new job or a major news event) to aid accurate recall.
- Decompose generic symptom memories by finding features that distinguish them from each other.
- Recall the symptom history in a retrograde fashion, beginning with the most recent event and working backwards.

The temporal dimension

Symptoms exhibit both short-term and long-term temporal variability. Some symptoms may be worse at particular times of the day or night, others such as headache, back pain or irritable bowel-related diarrhoea may be episodic and wax and wane in discrete time periods. Less than 4% of patients report that their symptoms are constant.

Over the longer term symptoms will also change irrespective of any treatment and this is a particular problem with new-onset symptoms. In a study of 500 adults presenting to a walk-in clinic in Washington DC with physical symptoms, 70% of patients improved within 2 weeks and nearly 90% got better within 3 months.[36] In an audit of patients visiting an emergency department for non-traumatic abdominal or flank pain, most improved within several days.[37] The long-term prognosis for patients presenting with a chief complaint of dizziness is also generally good: at least 28% recovered within 2 weeks; and of the remainder, more than half improved within a year.[38]

The skilled primary care-oriented diagnostician needs to know when to use a 'tincture of time' as opposed to rushing towards extensive and invasive investigations (*see* Chapter 3). Primary care diagnostics is also about sharing these concerns with the patient, a process that is facilitated by the continuity of care found in a number of primary care-oriented healthcare systems. In the UK, although each patient–doctor interaction may last only 10 minutes it seems that, over the course of 1 year, patients consult their general practitioner for an average of 47 minutes.

The other problem facing the primary care clinician is that they will encounter conditions and symptoms at a more evolutionary stage when the characteristics of symptoms are changing; by the time the patient reaches the ward or the specialist clinic the description of the symptom may have become more fixed and moreover

TABLE 4.11 Symptoms of meningitis in children

Symptom	Mean time to symptom(hours)	Children with meningitis who show symptom (%)
Fever	1	94
Irritability	4	67
Drowsiness	7	81
Abnormal skin colour	10	19
Cold hands and feet	12	43
Haemorrhagic rash	13	61
Neck pain or stiffness	13	35
Photophobia	15	28
Confusion or delirium	16	45

the patient will have had more time to reflect on their story. Melbye *et al.* examined the value of dyspnoea and chest pain in relation to the diagnosis of pneumonia. They noted that the illness duration had important effects on the validity of the symptoms.[39]

As a primary care clinician one of my greatest concerns has always been to avoid missing the diagnosis of meningitis. A few years ago I was called to see a child at an isolated farm who seemed to be a bit 'dopey' and who had a generalised, blotchy rash. The child had no neck stiffness, no photophobia and no purpura. Thankfully, I decided to give the child benzylpenicillin and send them into hospital. A florid purpuric rash appeared as they arrived on the hospital ward. In some recent work on the early symptoms of meningitis in children, it seems that the 'classical signs' often develop quite late (*see* Table 4.11).[40]

The environment

Symptom reporting is not divorced from the environment that the patient inhabits. Group health beliefs and attitudes may both discourage and encourage symptom reporting by emphasising the significance of some symptoms and yet playing down the importance of others. Cardol and colleagues have noted how the consultation patterns for headaches and abdominal pain seem to run in families.[41] In some areas where I have practised, vertigo and headaches can be particularly distressing not just due to the symptoms but because these symptoms appear to create worries about a possible brain tumour. Such beliefs seem to be held by families or communities and failing to address them can lead to considerable distress and unnecessary investigations. In contrast, and as discussed earlier, many cancer-related symptoms may be dismissed or ignored.

Social attitudes can also impact on symptom reporting. For example, Bluestein and Levin noted that women with wanted pregnancies were more likely than women with unwanted pregnancies to report amenorrhoea, breast tenderness and morning sickness.[42] This social acceptability bias must always be considered when we are dealing with symptoms that may be associated with socially sensitive problems such as sexually transmitted diseases, psychological problems, alcohol or drug abuse. Careful questioning may be required in such circumstances with the question being framed in a non-judgemental fashion. Social acceptability is discussed in greater detail in Chapter 5.

At one point in my career I undertook a series of locums in a number of different practices. No matter whether the practice was located in a fairly affluent area or in a relatively deprived one, the cleanliness of the premises seemed to bear a direct relationship to the magnitude of the clinical problems I encountered. Obviously this is merely a subjective impression but in a small study it was found that individuals rated their health as better (with fewer symptoms) when they were interviewed in a clean and well-maintained office compared to a dirty, over-heated laboratory with flickering lights and distracting noise. Although home visits are not as common as they used to be in British general practice, they may still sometimes have a valuable role in helping to understand a symptom by placing it in context.

GENERAL REFERENCES

- Armstrong BK, White E, Saracci R. *Principles of Exposure Measurement in Epidemiology.* Oxford: Oxford University Press, 1992.
- Barsky AJ. Forgetting, fabricating and telescoping: the instability of the medical history. *Arch Intern Med* 2002; **162**: 981–4.
- Jones R, Britten N, Culpepper L, *et al. Oxford Textbook of Primary Medical Care.* Oxford: Oxford University Press, 2003.
- McWhinney IR. *A Textbook of Family Medicine.* Oxford: Oxford University Press, 1997.
- Pendleton D, Schofield T, Tate P, *et al. The Consultation: an approach to learning and teaching.* Oxford: Oxford University Press, 1984.
- Stewart M, Brown JB, Weston WW, *et al. Patient-Centred Medicine: transforming the clinical method.* Oxford: Radcliffe Medical Press, 2003.

TEXT REFERENCES

1. Hippocrates. (Lloyd GER, editor) *Hippocratic Writings.* London: Penguin Books, 1978.
2. Kahwati LC, Haigler L, Rideout S. What is the best way to diagnose menopause? *J Fam Pract* 2005; **54**: 1000–2.
3. Bastian LA, Smoth CM, Nanda K. Is this woman perimenopausal? *JAMA* 2003; **289**: 895–902.
4. Richards D, Toop L, Chambers S, *et al.* Response to antibiotics of women with symptoms of urinary tract infection but negative dipstick urine test results: double blind randomised controlled trial. *BMJ* 2005; **331**: 143–6.

5. McGee S. *Evidence-Based Physical Diagnosis.* Philadelphia: WB Saunders, 2001.

6. Law M, Morris JK, Jordan R, *et al.* Headaches and the treatment of blood pressure: results from a meta-analysis of 94 randomised placebo-controlled trials with 24,000 participants. *Circulation* 2005; **112**: 2301–6.

7. Bass MJ, McWhinney IR, Dempsey IB, *et al.* Predictors of outcome in headache patients presenting to family practitioners – a one year prospective study. *Headache J* 1986; **26**: 285–90.

8. De Dombal FT. *Diagnosis of Acute Abdominal Pain.* Edinburgh: Churchill Livingstone, 1991.

9. Anderson MR, Klink K, Cohrssen A. Evaluation of vaginal complaints. *JAMA* 2004; **291**: 1368–79.

10. Wulff HR, Gotzsche PC. *Rational Diagnosis and Treatment: evidence-based clinical decision-making.* Oxford: Blackwell, 2000.

11. Walker RD. Knowledge of symptoms suggesting malignant disease among general practice patients. *J Roy Coll Gen Pract* 1982; **32**: 163–70.

12. Huygen FJA. *Family Medicine – the medical life history of families.* London: RCGP, 1990.

13. Banks MH, Beresford SAA, Morrell DC, *et al.* Factors influencing demand for primary medical care in women aged 20–44 years: a preliminary report. *Int J Epidemiol* 1975; **4**: 189–99.

14. Summerton N, Mann S, Rigby AS, *et al.* Patients with new onset haematuria: assessing the discriminant value of items of clinical information in relation to urological malignancies. *Brit J Gen Pract* 2002; **52**: 284–9.

15. Kroenke K, Price RK. Symptoms in the community: prevalence, classification and psychiatric comorbidity. *Arch Intern Med* 1993; **153**: 2474–80.

16. Kroenke K, Mangelsdorff D. Common symptoms in ambulatory care. *Am J Med* 1989; **86**: 262–6.

17. Buntinx F, Knockaert D, Bruyninckx R, *et al.* Chest pain in general practice or in the hospital emergency department: is it the same? *Family Practice* 2001; **18**: 586–9.

18. Mayou R, Farmer A. Functional somatic symptoms and syndromes. *BMJ* 2002; **325**: 265–8.

19. O'Malley PG, Jackson JL, Santoro J, *et al.* Antidepressant therapy for unexplained symptoms and symptom syndromes. *J Fam Pract* 1999; **48**: 980–90.

20. Kroenke K. Studying symptoms: sampling and measurement issues. *Ann Intern Med* 2001; **134**: 844–53.

21. Muris JW, Starmans R, Fijten GH. One-year prognosis of abdominal complaints in general practice: a prospective study of patients in whom no organic cause is found. *Brit J Gen Pract* 1996; **46**: 715–19.

22. Berger MY, Olde Hartman TC, van der Velden JJ, *et al.* Is biliary pain exclusively related to gallbladder stones? A controlled prospective study. *Brit J Gen Pract* 2004; **54**: 574–9.

23. Thiadens HA, de Bock GH, Dekker FW, *et al.* Identifying asthma and chronic obstructive pulmonary disease in patients with persistent cough presenting to general practitioners: descriptive study. *BMJ* 1998; **316**: 1286–90.

24. Summerton N, Mann S, Rigby AS, *et al.* New onset palpitations in general practice: assessing the discriminant value of items within the clinical history. *Family Practice* 2001; **18**: 383–92.

25. Fraser RC. *Clinical Method: a general practice approach*. Oxford: Butterworth-Heinemann, 1999.

26. Chen W, Woods SL, Puntillo KA. Gender differences in symptoms associated with acute myocardial infarction: a review of research. *Heart and Lung* 2005; **34**: 240–7.

27. Christos PJ, Oliveria SA, Berwick M, *et al.* Signs and symptoms of melanoma in older populations. *J Clin Epidemiol* 2000; **53**: 1044–53.

28. Funk M, Naum JB, Milner KA. Presentation and symptom predictors of coronary heart disease in patients with and without diabetes. *Am J Emerg Med* 2001; **19**: 482–7.

29. Bytzer P, Talley NJ, Leemon M, *et al.* Prevalence of gastrointestinal symptoms associated with diabetes mellitus: a population-based survey of 15,000 adults. *Arch Intern Med* 2001; **161**: 1989–96.

30. Patel P, Henry LL, Ganti AK, *et al.* Clinical course of lung cancer in patients with chronic kidney disease. *Lung Cancer* 2004; **43**: 297–300.

31. Colledge NR, Barr-Hamilton RM, Lewis SJ, *et al.* Evaluation of investigations to diagnose the cause of dizziness in elderly people: a community based controlled study. *BMJ* 1996; **313**: 788–92.

32. Sapira JD. *The Art and Science of Bedside Diagnosis*. Philadelphia: Williams & Wilkins, 1990.

33. Boyle CM. Difference between patients' and doctors' interpretation of some common medical terms. *BMJ* 1970; **2**: 286–9.

34. Cochrane AL, Chapman PJ. Observers' errors in taking medical histories. *Lancet* 1951; **1**: 1007–9.

35. Summerton N, Mann S, Sutton J, *et al.* Developing clinically relevant and reproducible symptom-defined populations for cancer diagnostic research in general practice using a community survey. *Family Practice* 2003; **20**: 340–6.

36. Kroenke K, Jackson JL. Outcome in general medical patients presenting with common symptoms: a prospective study with a 2-week and a 3-month follow-up. *Family Practice* 1998; **15**: 398–403.

37. Weiner JB, Nagurney JT, Brown DFM, *et al.* Duration of symptoms and follow-up patterns of patients discharged from the emergency department after presenting with abdominal or flank pain. *Family Practice* 2004; **21**: 314–16.

38. Kroenke K, Lucas CA, Rosenberg ML, *et al.* Causes of persistent dizziness: a prospective study of 100 patients in ambulatory care. *Ann Intern Med* 1992: **117**: 898–904.

39. Melbye H, Straume B, Assebo U, *et al.* The diagnosis of adult pneumonia in general practice. *Scand J Primary Health Care* 1988; **6**: 111–17.

40. Thompson MJ, Ninis N, Perera R, *et al.* Clinical recognition of meningococcal disease in children and adolescents. *Lancet* 2006; **367**: 397–403.

41. Cardol M, Vanden Bosch WJHM, Spreeuwenberg P, *et al.* All in the family: headaches and abdominal pain as indicators of consultation pattern in families. *Ann Fam Med* 2006; **4**: 506–11.

42. Bluestein D, Levin JS. Symptom reporting in wanted and unwanted pregnancies. *Family Medicine* 1991; **23**: 271–4.

CHAPTER 5

Past medical history

INTRODUCTION

Once we have established and assessed the nature of the patient's presenting problem, there is often a temptation to move straight on to examining the patient or
undertaking some preliminary investigations. However, the essence of primary care
diagnostics is to derive as much information as possible from the patient. Even
once they have described and been questioned about their symptoms, the patient
still has useful diagnostic data to offer in terms of their previous healthcare, health
behaviours, social, occupational and family history.

The additional information in the past medical history may have a particularly significant place in diagnostic decision making when there are some concerns about the validity or the reliability of the symptom(s). For example, in a
study of 400 patients with dyspepsia consulting their general practitioner, it was
concluded that the symptom-based diagnoses were unreliable in distinguishing
between reflux disease, functional diseases and organic conditions such as gall-
stones, peptic ulceration and malignancy. The authors suggested that, in selecting patients for gastroscopy, more weight should be attached to other features
such as the patient's age, their use of non-steroidal anti-inflammatory drugs
(NSAIDs) and a history of previous peptic ulceration.[1] Questioning patients
about NSAID and aspirin use (both prescribed and purchased over-the-counter)
is frequently neglected.

In this chapter three aspects of the medical history are focused on which can
have a particular bearing on primary care diagnostics: previous healthcare, health
behaviour and the family history. The chapter concludes with an assessment of the
diagnosis of migraine using information derived solely from the patient's symptoms and their past medical history.

PREVIOUS HEALTHCARE

In seeking to harness the patient's previous healthcare history for diagnostic
purposes, two issues need to be considered - predictive validity and concurrent validity.

Predictive validity

Back pain

Back pain is a common problem presenting to primary care clinicians. Patients are often concerned about the cause of the pain but there is a persisting controversy regarding the initial evaluation of such patients. Lumbar-spine films are frequently obtained but have a low yield, may be misleading, represent a significant dose of radiation and are expensive. It has been suggested that features in the history and examination could be utilised in order to allow the more selective use of radiology without missing serious underlying diseases.

Deyo and Diehl evaluated nearly 2000 walk-in patients in a public hospital in the US with a chief complaint of back pain.[2] By comparing features about the patients' healthcare history, personal characteristics, symptoms and clinical examination against a diagnostic reference standard, positive likelihood ratios were calculated for the diagnosis of cancer. The information is shown in Table 5.1.

As Table 5.1 shows, the magnitude of the likelihood ratio diminishes as we move down the table from features in the previous healthcare history, personal characteristics, to symptoms and, finally, to some aspects of the clinical examination. Simple investigations were also helpful: an ESR (erythrocyte sedimentation rate) > 20 mm/hr provided a positive likelihood ratio of 2.4 and an ESR > 50 a positive likelihood ratio of 19.2. The authors concluded that combining historical features and ESR results could have reduced radiograph utilisation to just 22% of subjects, while recommending a radiograph for every cancer patient. Moreover, the work could also suggest which patients with negative radiographic findings require further investigation.

TABLE 5.1 Positive likelihood ratios for back pain and cancer diagnosis

Clinical feature	Positive likelihood ratio
Previous healthcare history:	
previous history of cancer	14.7
sought medical care in last month, not improving	3.0
Personal characteristics:	
age > 50 years	2.7
Symptoms:	
unexplained weight loss	2.7
duration of episode > 1 month	2.6
insidious onset	1.1
Clinical examination:	
muscle spasm	0.5
spine tenderness	0.4

Palpitations

Palpitations are another symptom where information from the previous healthcare history can be useful in distinguishing patients with clinically significant arrhythmias from those without. Over a 2-year period, Zwietering *et al.* took a structured history from 762 patients with new complaints possibly related to arrhythmias.[3] These included all patients attending their general practitioner because of palpitations, together with a few others consulting their GP about dyspnoea, faintness, angina pectoris, fatigue, collapse and other symptoms if the GP considered an arrhythmia as a possible cause of the complaints. This information was compared against that derived from a transtelephonic electrocardiogram (the reference standard).

Table 5.2 details those features in the past history that were either positively or negatively associated with clinically relevant arrhythmias. For the positive associations the value of the odds ratio represents the likelihood of a clinically significant arrhythmia. Conversely, for the negative associations more importance is attached to the smaller odds ratios as they represent a very low likelihood of a clinically significant arrhythmia.

Pattern of attendance

In relation to cancer diagnosis, aside from the use of symptoms (e.g. change in bowel habit or rectal bleeding for colorectal cancer diagnosis), it has been suggested that certain pieces of clinical information more readily and uniquely available in primary care settings such as changes in a patient's behaviour may have significant weights of evidence in assisting the diagnosis of malignancy. Moreover, it may even be possible to quantify such behavioural changes by looking at alterations in, perhaps, smoking

TABLE 5.2 Previous healthcare history and significant arrhythmias

Features in previous healthcare history	Odds ratio
Positive associations:	
known hypertension	1.9
known arrhythmias	8.5
known other cardiovascular disease	3.3
known other diseases	1.7
using cardiovascular medications	5.8
using diuretics	3.7
Negative associations:	
known frequent psychosomatic complaints	0.2
frequent attender	0.4
using CNS medication	0.4

status, consultation patterns (a measure of healthcare-seeking behaviour), the use of over-the-counter medications or accompanied surgery attendances.

There is particularly a strong tradition within British general practice that patients who visit their general practitioner with a new problem after a long period of non-attendance are more likely to have a cancer. Using a case-control study design we attempted to test this hypothesis by examining a patient's consultation pattern for the 3 years leading up to the diagnosis of an internal malignancy within the context of my own general practice.[4] Using a combination of matching, consultation sub-classification and conditional logistic regression, account was taken of the major confounders affecting consultation rates.

Our work revealed that, in general, the odds of cancer rose in tandem with increases in the average time between new consultations. This trend reached statistical significance for all breast cancers and persisted after adjustment for occupation, smoking and marital status as well as after the exclusion of patients identified by routine screening.

Over the years a lot of work has been undertaken in seeking to understand the determinants of consultation. The reasons why a patient with, for example, cancer-related dyspepsia delays attending are many and various and remain only partially understood. It is certainly the case that patients with dyspepsia who choose to consult have, in general, more frequent and severe symptoms. However, the decision to see a physician is not based simply on the presence or absence of medical problems: for example, fear of cancer may either facilitate or retard consultation. Our preliminary work is different in that, rather than trying to simply explain the consultation pattern, we sought to harness it as a tool to assist with cancer diagnosis.

In relation to recognition of other important conditions such as parasuicide risk or urinary tract infections in children it seems that here too the patient's pattern of attendance may have some potential diagnostic value. Prior to any parasuicidal attempt patients attend more frequently than their peers and the consultation rate accelerates up until the time of the attempt.[5] Compared to a group of matched controls, children eventually diagnosed with urinary tract infections had a mean 2.94 additional GP visits (or 21% more visits) in the 2.5 years prior to the definitive diagnosis of their first urinary tract infection.[6] In patients with chest problems, a duration of illness less than 24 hours before consulting their general practitioner was the variable in the history with the highest likelihood ratio for pneumonia diagnosis (*see* Table 5.3).[7]

TABLE 5.3 Promptness of consulting and pneumonia diagnosis

Duration of illness before consulting	Likelihood ratio
< 1 day	13.5
< 4 days	2.0
> 7 days	0.5

In contrast, fever only provided a likelihood ratio of 1.2, bloody sputum 2.3, yellow sputum 0.9, chest pain 1.3 and chills 1.3.

Concurrent validity

A few years ago my colleagues and I undertook a study examining previous clinical encounters amongst patients undergoing barium enemas. A particular interest was the frequency of rectal examination and one of the most surprising results was the level of disagreement between doctors and patients. Some patients denied having had a rectal examination whereas the doctor assured us that they had and, even more bizarrely, a number of patients indicated that they had undergone a rectal examination when the general practitioner was quite confident that this was not the case.[8]

As has been discussed already in Chapter 4, whatever element of the history we are seeking to use for diagnostic purposes, misunderstandings, forgetfulness, cognitive problems such as telescoping and recomposition, and social acceptability biases all need to be taken into account. A good example of misunderstanding occurs in osteoarthritis. In a study of the medical records in two UK general practices, the level of agreement between the doctors' coding of osteoarthritis and patients' use of the term osteoarthritis was no greater than would be expected by chance alone.[9] Telescoping effects, whereby past events are remembered as if they occurred closer to the present time than was actually the case, have been reported in relation to dates of the last tetanus booster and fractures in perimenopausal women.[10] It also seems that women report more cervical smears over the preceding five years than their medical records suggest and often state that their last smear is more recent than laboratory records indicate. Recomposition, in which similar events are brought together as a single event, has been demonstrated for women with long mammography histories in comparison with younger women or women with less mammography experience.[11]

There is a bias associated with reporting psychological or sexual issues. With this in mind it is interesting to note that forgetting prior episodes of depression is common: of those with a diagnosis of depression up to age 21, only 44% recalled a key symptom when they were re-questioned several years later.[12] In a survey of past surgical history no male patients admitted to genito-urinary surgery unless directly questioned.[13]

Another specific cognitive bias that may impact on a patient's description of their previous medical care is the halo effect. This results in one discrete event (e.g. a success or a failure) exerting undue influence (positively or negatively) on the patient's description and recall of *all their care* by a specific clinician or hospital. A competent doctor who, through no fault of his own, misses a critical diagnosis may be more generally remembered in a particularly bad light.

In order to assess the concurrent validity of the past medical history, patients attending general ophthalmology outpatient clinics in Boston, US, were questioned about common chronic diseases and some associated treatments.[14] These data were compared against other sources of information in order to calculate sensitivities (a measure of under-reporting) and specificities (a measure of over-reporting) (*see* Table 5.4).

Coronary heart disease, cancer and the use of steroids were particularly likely to be under-reported. Arthritis and aspirin use exhibit both over-reporting and under-reporting; those with less than 12 years of education were more likely to over-report a history of arthritis and yet under-report regular aspirin use.

Other studies of self-reported cancer and heart disease histories have confirmed these findings. Comparing cancer histories with cancer registry data has also revealed that, whereas the overall sensitivity of cancer reporting is 79%, doctors should have considerably more confidence in a history of breast (sensitivity 91%), prostate (sensitivity 90%) and lung (sensitivity 90%) cancers as opposed to melanoma (sensitivity 53%).[15] Lower sensitivity was also found for cancer reports in individuals over the age of 70 years, current smokers and those who did not graduate from high school. This effect of education is also seen in relation to fracture reporting in older women, which was more accurate amongst individuals with a college education.

For some conditions there appears to be confusion amongst patients with a closely related condition thereby lowering the reported sensitivity. For example, acute myocardial infarction (reported sensitivity 60%) may not be clearly distinguished from angina; and rectal cancer (reported sensitivity 16%) might simply not be seen as any different from colon cancer.[16] Confusion may also occur if the treatment of malignant, pre-malignant and benign conditions is similar (e.g. for transurethral resection of the prostate or total abdominal hysterectomy). Such factors should be borne in mind when taking a history; for example in seeking to

TABLE 5.4 Sensitivity and specificity of reported elements in the past history

Medical history reported	Sensitivity (i.e. proportion answering 'yes' if disease was present) (%)	Specificity (i.e. proportion answering 'no' if disease was absent) (%)
Arthritis	75	66
Coronary heart disease	64	96
Hypertension	91	88
Diabetes	84	97
Cancer	71	89
Use of oral hypoglycaemic	78	98
Use of regular aspirin	73	70
Use or oral steroids	66	96
Use of anti-hypertensives	88	89

identify patients with ischaemic heart disease, episodes of angina and myocardial infarcts should be specifically and separately enquired about.

A serious, novel or unique event in the previous medical history is more likely to be remembered consistently and reliably. For fractures anatomical site and severity appear to aid recall; reports of major fractures such as the hip and wrist are considerably more reliable than reports of finger, toe and rib fractures.[16] Surgery performed in childhood (e.g. tonsillectomy) or regarded as 'minor' (e.g. dental extractions) is also likely to be very poorly remembered. It is also important to be aware that different interviewers can elicit different information.[13] In the study of English coal miners referred to in Chapter 4 a history of pneumonia was uncovered in only under 12% of patients by one doctor but in over 15% by another.[17]

Enhancing concurrent validity

In relation to past medication use it seems that specific questioning may be more productive then open-ended questioning. Two studies have revealed that medication use was more likely to be recalled accurately if patients were asked about specific drugs. Visual aids may also help and women's recall of the name and the dose of hormone-replacement therapy can be improved by using photographs of preparations. In dating past medical events, access to a calendar can be very helpful and some patients even keep personal records that can supplement the information provided in the course of the medical interview.

Information may also be obtained from the individual's existing medical records but problems can occur due to time gaps, missing information, ambiguities or inconstancies. I recently encountered a 50-year-old man who had been labelled as having a stroke; after a number of telephone calls and a discussion with his original neurologist, the true diagnosis turned out to be migraine! Unfortunately, symptoms, risk factors or personal information are all too often poorly and inconsistently recorded. Amongst the records of a group of cancer patients, 15% had missing information on smoking, 25% on alcohol consumption and 36% on occupation.

It has been suggested that reports from relatives and friends can be helpful in improving the concurrent validity of the past healthcare history and such information may also be particularly useful if the patient is demented or a minor. Certainly patients and their next-of-kin showed similar levels of agreement in reporting the use of prescription medicines.[18] However, the agreement between patients and their relatives was much poorer when it came to over-the-counter medicines such as antacids, antihistamines and analgesics. There may also be a gap in information quality; for example, in one study although husbands were able to accurately report whether their wife was a current or past user of oral contraceptives, most were unable to name the brand of the oral contraceptive or to give an estimate of the duration of use.[19] Similarly, although relatives can provide reliable information on an older woman's history of childbirth, using such proxy respondents for non-obstetric surgery may result in substantial under-reporting.[20] There is also a tendency for proxies to over-estimate specific behaviours such as cigarette consumption.

In examining the information provided by different proxies it seems that, in general, close relatives – spouse, sibling, parent or child – usually provide more complete data than other proxy respondents. In obtaining information on psychiatric disorders the degree of inter-informant reproducibility varied from a kappa of 0.58 (moderate agreement) for dementia, 0.41 (moderate agreement) for alcoholism, 0.26 (slight agreement) for depression to 0.19 (poor agreement) for anxiety disorders. Furthermore, the spouse or child will generally be able to provide more information about the subject's adult life, while a parent or sibling is likely to know more about the subject's childhood or young adult life.

Despite these rather unexciting findings in relation to the past medical history I still consider that relatives have a key diagnostic role. Even before they speak I attach some possible diagnostic significance to their actual attendance with the patient and I would even suggest that there might be a 'dose–response' effect with the number of relatives attending being proportional to the seriousness of the condition! Furthermore, although 'doctor-centred' research indicates that questioning relatives about specific memory impairments can be inaccurate in 40% of cases, family members may be able to provide key information on more 'patient and family oriented' measures such as day-to-day functioning and behaviour. Early on in the dementing process many relatives often mention that something is going wrong and that the patient is requiring an increasing level of support.

HEALTH BEHAVIOUR

Understanding a patient's health behaviours is important in seeking to reach a diagnosis. Smoking, sexual practices and alcohol consumption can be associated with a number of symptoms and illnesses. Unfortunately patients may over-report what they consider to be socially desirable behaviours and yet under-report apparently socially undesirable behaviours. Whenever I encounter a child with a wheezy chest I always make a point of asking the parents about their smoking habits. Even if the child's clothes reek of smoke the parents still indicate (often quite forcefully) that they *always* smoke outside the house. However, after several years of driving around the towns and villages of Yorkshire on home visits I am yet to encounter a single individual smoking out in their garden on a cold day!

Eliciting information about certain sexual behaviours may be more difficult if the patient is accompanied by a child and/or their spouse and/or the doctor is of the opposite sex. It also takes more skilled questioning to extract information about, for example, sexual activity, alcohol consumption or drug use. Suggested approaches include the use of words familiar to the patient, open-ended questioning, avoiding the issue at the beginning of the interview and a longer (and non-threatening) introduction to a question, e.g. 'occasionally people drink a little too much and become intoxicated [or an equivalent word that may be more meaningful to the patient than "intoxicated"]. In the past year, how often … ?'. One (albeit rather less honest) mechanism is the use of 'bogus testing' whereby the individual is led to believe that a parallel 'laboratory test' is being used to assess the accuracy of their responses. Certainly such an approach has been applied successfully to enhance the accuracy of the reporting of alcohol, drug and cigarette use.

Personally I find individuals who smoke much easier to spot than patients who are abusing alcohol. Recently I encountered a patient with peripheral paraesthesia who I carefully examined and arranged a battery of investigations. However, I felt rather shame-faced when a newly qualified colleague subsequently identified that the patient was consuming over 70 units of alcohol per week. Unfortunately I am not alone: in a group of American family doctors only 19% were able to correctly diagnose an alcohol problem presented in computer simulations. Similarly, amongst Australian general practitioners, less than 28% of heavy drinkers were identified. Ironically problem drinkers are actually more likely to consult a doctor: in France it was discovered that 16% of patients consulting their general practitioner had an alcohol problem, 27% of men and 5% of women.[21]

The other important factor about alcohol consumption is that, if recognised, simple brief interventions which can be practised in primary care settings are remarkably effective.

There is a need to have a high index of suspicion about alcohol abuse when confronted with a broad range of often vague symptoms, e.g. gastrointestinal, neurological and psychological. It is now generally agreed that drinking becomes hazardous at above 21 units weekly for men and 14 units weekly for women. However, quantifying the number of units can be tricky and I find the data in Table 5.5 particularly helpful.[22]

There is a need for care when trying to assess consumption, as in our own ongoing research we have discovered that comparing 'food and drink' diaries with simple stated consumption in a consultation reveals consistent under-reporting. In the context of an interview it also seems that more accuracy can be achieved by enquiring about alcohol in a few different ways in the middle of an interview rather than at the beginning or at the end. The time frame is also important; once I estimated a patient's alcohol consumption at 15 units, which seemed quite reasonable. However, I subsequently realised that the patient had been thinking in terms of a day rather than a week!

In determining whether a patient is actually abusing alcohol, additional information is required. To assist with this a number of questionnaires (e.g. CAGE) are available as well as some laboratory tests (e.g. mean cell volume [MCV] and gamma glutamyl transferase [GGT]). The brevity of the CAGE questionnaire (see Box 5.1) and its non-intimidating approach makes it particularly applicable to primary care settings.[22]

TABLE 5.5 Alcohol units for alcoholic drinks

Alcoholic drink	Measure	Alcohol (unit)
Beers, lagers, cider	1 pint	2
	1 can	1.5
Low alcohol beers, lagers, cider	1 pint	0.6
	1 can	0.5
Strong beers, lagers, cider	1 pint	3
	1 can	2
Table wine	1 glass	1
	1 bottle (75 cl)	8
Sherry	1 standard small measure	1
	1 bottle	13
Spirits	1 standard measure	1.5
	1 bottle	30
'Alco-pops'	1 bottle	1.5

Box 5.1 CAGE questionnaire

Alcohol dependence is stated to be likely if the patient gives two or more positive answers to the following questions.
- Have you ever felt you should Cut down your drinking?
- Have people Annoyed you by criticising your drinking?
- Have you ever felt bad or Guilty about your drinking?
- Have you ever had a drink first thing in the morning to steady your nerves or get rid of a hangover (Eye-opener)?

In research conducted within some general practices in Belgium, sensitivities, specificities and likelihood ratios were identified for the CAGE questionnaire and the blood tests by comparison against reference standard criteria from the *Diagnostic and Statistical Manual of Mental Disorders*.[23] The results are shown in Table 5.6.

Thus the CAGE questions have better discriminant properties than either of the blood tests. Moreover, other work has demonstrated that the questionnaire can be similarly helpful in identifying individuals in other settings aside from European general practice. Examples include American Indians, walk-in centres, accident and emergency departments and Latinos living in the United States.

TABLE 5.6 Testing for alcohol abuse or dependence

'Test'	Sensitivity (%)	Specificity (%)	Positive likelihood ratio
CAGE (men)	62	81	3.3
CAGE (women)	55	92	6.9
MCV (men)	39	75	1.6
MCV (women)	41	79	2.0
GGT (men)	7	75	1.4
GGT (women)	7	92	0.8

Despite all this, a number of textbooks written by specialists for consumption by generalists still emphasise the diagnostic value of blood testing; this is another example of where valuable information that can obtained from the patient is being ignored.

FAMILY HISTORY

One of the cardinal features that differentiates primary care medicine from other clinical specialties is that primary care physicians remain generalists providing comprehensive care to patients in a holistic manner. The term 'family practice' used in some countries further emphasises that primary care physicians often care for family units and there are strong arguments in favour of knowing the nature of the family in dealing with an individual patient's problems.

In recent years knowledge about genetic influences on health has advanced rapidly and it is becoming increasingly clear that the majority of common and important conditions have a hereditary component. For example, individuals with a family history of cancer of the large bowel, breast, uterus or ovary face an increased risk of developing the same type of cancer themselves. Unfortunately the link between health and family membership is far from straightforward. There are a number of possible influences of the family on health aside from the genes such as living conditions, lifestyle (including health-related behaviours such as smoking and alcohol consumption), healthcare-seeking behaviour and the spread of communicable disease. Some symptoms such as headaches may have a familial clustering due to genetic influences but the link may also be related to social, psychological or even environmental (e.g. carbon monoxide poisoning) factors. Genetic disorders are also not easy to understand due to their multifactorial nature as well as their different degrees of penetrance. The relative risk of an individual having asthma, osteoporosis or schizophrenia is 2.6, 3.0 and 8.6 respectively if their sibling has the specified condition.

In 1997 we conducted a survey of family history taking amongst a sample of UK general practitioners.[24] The results revealed that, in addition to routinely recording

TABLE 5.7 Routine family history enquiries.

Condition	Practitioners stating that the condition was routinely enquired about on first registration (%)
Thyroid disease	20.8
Breast cancer	48.4
Rheumatoid disease	21.4
Coronary heart disease	94.3
Colon/rectal cancer	30.7

information about family history (*see* Table 5.7), 29% of the respondents indicated that they often or very often enquired about family medical history during a routine consultation.

Furthermore, in response to the question 'do you feel that knowing the family medical history helps you to reach a decision about …?' the responses shown in Table 5.8 were obtained.

The majority of the general practitioners who responded to this survey felt that knowing the family medical history would assist them in reaching a number of important medical decisions. Personally I know that I routinely ask about a family history of asthma in children with chest complaints and a family history of migraine when consulted by a patient with a possible migraine headache. Others have suggested that in children with headaches, an *absence* of a family history of migraine should be promoted as a strong indicator for neuroimaging. However, if the family history is being used as a diagnostic/decision-making tool we need to be confident about its validity and reliability.

TABLE 5.8 Does using the family medical history aid decision making in diagnosis?

Decision made	Practitioners stating likely or very likely to the use of the family medical history as an aid to decision making (%)
Ordering thyroid function test	57.8
Arranging investigations for rheumatoid disease	55.5
Checking a patient's cholesterol	92.1
Referral with a breast lump in a patient under 35	77.1
Referral for investigations in a patient under 50 with rectal bleeding	77.1
Referral for investigations in a patient under 50 with a persistent change in bowel habit	75.1

By means of a systematic review of the literature, my colleagues and I identified studies that sought to assess the accuracy of the cancer family history with a particular emphasis on breast and colorectal cancers (*see* Table 5.9).

From this review, it is clear that we should have greater confidence in cancer family history reports by first-degree relatives, especially if they are younger and female. This enhanced accuracy applies to both the presence of cancers in relatives in addition to their age of onset. Age at diagnosis is particularly important as patients developing cancer younger than expected increases the possibility of a hereditary component. Other work in relation to cardiovascular disease has also confirmed the enhanced validity of information derived from first-degree relatives.

Breast and colon cancer family histories exhibit some false reporting but, in general, it seems that false-negative cancer family history reporting is much more likely with endometrial cancers (sensitivity 29%), central nervous system tumours and haematological malignancies. Cancers that are frequently over-reported in relatives (false positives) include melanoma and non-colonic gastrointestinal malignancies.

For most of the reports identified in our systematic review there may be some concerns that the method by which the family histories were extracted is not applicable to primary care. We sought to address this issue ourselves by comparing the information contained in general practitioner referral letters with that obtained by a consultant in clinical genetics for patients referred to a clinic in Yorkshire. Our findings supported the conclusions from the systematic review, but there were some missing data as, unfortunately, general practitioners only reported age at diagnosis in one-quarter of cases.

The best mechanism to extract an accurate family history from patients in the context of the brief encounters in primary care remains a conundrum. As a comprehensive family history assessment can take up to 30 minutes, a number of alternative approaches have been suggested.

- Using self-completed patient paper questionnaires that the patient can even take home to discuss with other family members.
- Using computerised genograms.
- Inviting patients to attend a specific 'family history assessment' session.

ESTIMATING A POST-HISTORY PROBABILITY

In Chapter 3 I set out a framework for Bayesian decision making based on the formula:

$$\text{posterior odds} = \text{likelihood ratio} \times \text{prior odds}$$

In terms of probabilities I also detailed a sequence to assist with the understanding of diagnostic processing.

TABLE 5.9 Cancer family histories

Author	Year	Setting for family history assessment	Subjects	Method of family history assessment	Reference standard	Results
Love, Evans and Josten[25]	1985	University of Wisconsin, USA. Cancer prevention clinic	• 121 consecutive patients • Self-referred with more than one first- or second-degree relative identified as having cancer • 87% female • Mean age 40 (range 23–75)	Comprehensive questionnaire on family history, age at diagnosis and type of cancers in first-, second-, and third-degree relatives	Confirming medical records on relatives – i.e. pathology and operative reports, hospital admission and discharge summaries, death certificates and autopsy reports	• For 216 cases of cancer in 180 first-degree relatives, the primary cancer site was correctly identified in 83% of the cases • For second- and third-degree relatives, the histories of primary cancer were accurate in 71% of the cases • Accuracy rates were 91% and 89% for breast and colon cancers, respectively • False reports were more likely for third- and second-degree relatives (8.2% and 5.7%) than for first-degree relatives (3.2%)
Napier, Metzner and Johnson[26]	1972	Tecumseh County, USA. Community Health Study	9159 persons, the majority of whom (93%) lived in the Tecumseh study area	As part of a lifetime medical history collected by staff of trained lay interviewers particularly focusing on the cause of death in first-degree relatives	Death certificates for relatives dying after 1940	• Focusing on first-degree relatives of subjects; 274 were stated to have a family history of cancer and 228 of these were confirmed (a concurrence rate of 83%)

Kerber and Slattery[27]	1997	Diet, activity and reproduction on colon cancer study (DARCC), Utah	• 125 colon cancer cases and 206 controls in DARCC study • Age 30–79	Computer-supported interviewing focusing on detailed questions about each relative in sequence	Genealogic and cancer information contained in the Utah population database	• 83% sensitivities were obtained for subject reports of breast cancer; 73% for colorectal • Higher sensitivities were observed among younger subjects than older subjects; females reported family histories of cancer only slightly better than males • Educational status did not have a consistent effect on the accuracy of reporting
Theis, Boyd, Lockwood et al.[28]	1994	Princess Margaret Hospital, Toronto	• 165 breast cancer patients without brain metastases • Age 31–70 (mean age 52) • Hospital records indicated at least one first-degree relative with breast cancer • Subjects were of above average educational attainment	Mailed questionnaire subsequently supplemented by a standard family history interview	Contact with relatives combined with hospital, cancer registry or death records	• There was agreement with the reference standard for 94% of reports on first-degree relatives and 88% on second-degree relatives • Cancer site accuracy was greater in the case of first-degree relatives (94% compared to 72%) • Age at diagnosis was more accurate in the case of first-degree relatives (90% compared to 59%) • There was one false-positive report

(Continued)

TABLE 5.9 Cancer family histories (*Continued*)

Author	Year	Setting for family history assessment	Subjects	Method of family history assessment	Reference standard	Results
Floderus, Barlow and Mack[29]	1990	Sweden: population-based Swedish twin registry	115 pairs of twins in which one in the pair had suffered breast cancer (86 cases and 83 co-twins)	3 to 4-hour personal interview by nurses including questions about the occurrence of cancer amongst first- and second-degree relatives	• No reference standard • Looked at agreement between twins	• For all cancers there was agreement about 129 cases, another 48 cancers were mentioned only by the case twin and another 55 only by the co-twin (odds ratio = 1.14) • For breast cancer there was agreement about 22 events, another 12 cases were provided by the cancer twin and four by the co-twin (odds ratio = 1.48)
Douglas, O'Dair, Robinson et al.[30]	1999	Newcastle-upon-Tyne and St Mary's Hospital, Manchester (genetics clinics)	• Retrospective study of 595 case notes (400 from Newcastle, 195 from Manchester) of patients attending cancer family history clinics • No demographic data available, although authors comment that the majority were women	Family history assessment in a specialist cancer family history clinic	Verification of reported family history sought through death certificates, medical notes, histopathology and cancer registries	• Reported abdominal malignancies (bowel, ovary, endometrial, pancreas and prostate) were accurate in 80%, whereas 95% of reported breast cancers were accurate • Reports of cancers were accurate in 90% of first-degree relatives and 80% of second-degree relatives

Ward et al.[31]		Royal Brisbane Hospital, Brisbane, Australia	• 237 patients (74 cases and 163 controls) • Aged between 28 and 74 years (median 60 years) • Had undergone colonoscopy at Royal Brisbane Hospital (1980–1985) for bowel symptoms	• Detailed postal questionnaire focusing on colorectal cancer in first-degree relatives • Relatives, doctors and hospital reports and death certificates	• 77% of positive family histories were confirmed • 98% of negative family histories (i.e. no positive relatives) were correct • Sensitivity of self-reported family history was estimated to be 87% amongst cases and 82% amongst controls • Specificity was estimated to be 97% in both cases and controls • Accuracy of positive reports was higher amongst women
Kee and Collins[32]	1991	Northern Ireland; Community	• 205 patients aged < 55 years • Histological diagnosis of colorectal cancer made between 1976 and 1978 (NB: next of kin contacted if patient deceased)	Home interview of surviving patient or next of kin • Contacts with general practitioners in Northern Ireland for relatives resident there • Postal survey of first-degree relatives living outside Northern Ireland • Information checked with hospital records and cancer registration records	• 96% of the cases of cancer in first-degree relatives were verified

(Continued)

TABLE 5.9 Cancer family histories (*Continued*)

Author	Year	Setting for family history assessment	Subjects	Method of family history assessment	Reference standard	Results
Glanz, Grove, Le March and et al.[33]	1999	Hawaii, USA; Community	• 274 siblings and 152 children (out of a pool of 553 first-degree relatives) • 49.3% male • Mean age 50 (19–84)	• Mailed survey to relatives of colorectal cancer patients • The survey enquired whether a parent and/ or a sibling had been diagnosed as having cancer of the colon or other cancers	Previously confirmed histological diagnosis of colorectal cancer	• 25.4% of respondents reported (wrongly) having no first-degree relatives with colon cancer • Most significant predictor in multivariate analysis of awareness of a relative's colorectal cancer was the stage at diagnosis (i.e. disseminated disease is associated with greater awareness): odds ratio 7.48 compared to 20.15 • Females (odds ratio 1.64) and those with greater knowledge of colorectal cancer (odds ratio 1.17) were more aware about the family history
Winter, Wiesner, Finnegan et al.[34]	1996	Minnesota, USA; Community	• 376 relatives of 160 breast cancer patients (out of a pool of 544 breast cancer families) • Mean age 66 years • 79% female	Telephone interview (using open-ended question to 'assess each contact's prior knowledge of his or her family history of breast cancer')	Previously confirmed breast cancer	• 26% of participants were unaware of their family history • First-degree relatives were more aware (98%) than were second-degree relatives (73%) • Female relatives were more aware of their breast cancer family history than their male counterparts (77% compared to 63%)

| Parent, Ghadirian, Lacroix et al.[35] | 1995 | University of Montreal, Canada. Participants in a study of nutritional factors and breast cancer | • 68 women with breast cancer (out of a pool of 414 patients with cancer)
 • 37 women without breast cancer (out of a pool of 429 controls)
 • Reporting at least one first-degree relative affected by cancer
 • Mean age 59 years (range 30–79 years) | Face to face interview focusing on relatives affected with *any* type of cancer using simple questions 'that would resemble those used in a medical setting', i.e. name of affected relative, cancer site and age at diagnosis | • Pathological confirmation sought only for first-degree relatives reportedly affected with breast cancer
 • No death certificates sought | • The presence of breast cancer was verified for 90.5% of the reports by affected patients (i.e. 9.5% false-positive) and 97% of the reports by unaffected patients (i.e. 3% false-negative)
 • One-third of the study participants reported the exact age at diagnosis for their relatives and 89% of reports were correct within 5 years
 • Cancer patients over the age of 70 years made large errors when reporting age at diagnosis for their relatives |

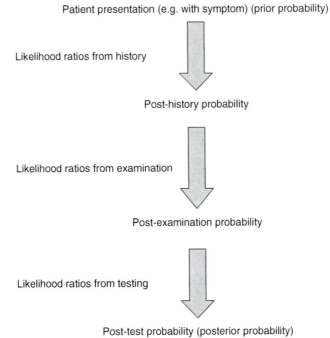

Patient presentation (e.g. with symptom) (prior probability)

Likelihood ratios from history

Post-history probability

Likelihood ratios from examination

Post-examination probability

Likelihood ratios from testing

Post-test probability (posterior probability)

Migraine serves as a model for the role of the input derived directly from the patient in moving from the prior probability to a post-history probability. Migraine diagnosis seems to be a particular problem in primary care and is frequently misdiagnosed or inappropriately treated. For example, in a study in the US, 88% of patients with a history of so-called 'sinus' headache were discovered to be suffering from migraine.[36]

The prior probability of migraine can be obtained from a study of the final diagnoses amongst a group of 265 patients presenting to family physicians with a new complaint of headache.[37] Of these patients, 5.3% eventually turned out to have migraine (i.e. the prior probability of migraine in patients presenting to primary care clinicians with new-onset headache is 5.3%).

Smetana has also collected together information on the positive and negative likelihood ratios (predictive of migraine) amongst patients with primary headaches (*see* Table 5.10).[38]

In a patient with a new-onset unilateral (LR+ 3.1) headache and nausea (LR+ 23.2), there are two approaches to integrating this information with the prior probability.

- **Approach 1:** Multiply together the two positive likelihood ratios (71.9) and place a ruler on the nomogram in Figure 5.1 linking the prior probability of 5.3%, through the likelihood ratio product (71.9) to the posterior (or in this case the post-history) probability. The result is a probability of approximately 80%.

TABLE 5.10 Likelihood ratios for migraine

Symptom or feature in medical history	Positive likelihood ratio (LR+)	Negative likelihood ratio (LR–)
Nausea	23.2	0.19
Photophobia	6.0	0.24
Phonophobia	5.2	0.38
Exacerbated by physical activity	3.7	0.24
Unilateral	3.1	0.43
Throbs or pulsates	3.3	0.32
Duration 4-24 hours	1.7	0.64
Precipitated by chocolate	4.6	0.82
Precipitated by cheese	4.9	0.68
Precipitated by alcohol	1.3	0.91
Family history of migraine	5.0	0.47
Personal history of childhood vomiting attacks	2.4	0.79

- **Approach 2:** Calculate the post-history probability using odds and the following formula.

post-history odds = likelihood ratio (for unilateral headache) × likelihood ratio (for nausea) × prior odds

- Convert the prior probability to odds using odds
  = probability/1– probability (i.e. odds = 0.056).
- Multiply the odds by the likelihood ratio product (i.e. 0.056 × 71.9) = 4.03.
- Convert back to probabilities using probability
  = odds/1 + odds (i.e.4.03/5.03) = 80%.

Thus using either of the approaches it is clear that some selected information derived from the history alone can have quite a dramatic effect on the disease probability. Eighty per cent is also probably well above the action threshold discussed in Chapter 3. However, the following additional issues also need to be borne in mind:
- The independence of likelihood ratios (*see* Chapter 6).
- The internal and external validity of the research study used to derive the likelihood ratios (*see* Chapter 8).
- The inter- and intra-observer reproducibility and the concurrent validity of the clinical indicants (*see* Chapter 3).

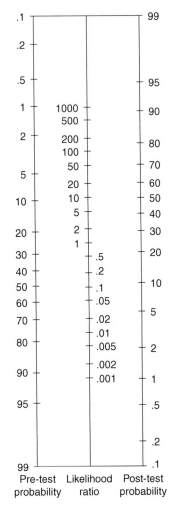

FIGURE 5.1 The Fagan Likelihood Ratio nomogram. Adapted with permission from Fagan TJ. Nomogram for Bayes' Theorem. *N Engl J Med* 1975; **293**: 257. © Massachusetts Medical Society. All rights reserved.

GENERAL REFERENCES

- Armstrong BK, White E, Saracci R. *Principles of Exposure Measurement in Epidemiology*. Oxford: Oxford University Press, 1992.
- Barsky AJ. Forgetting, fabricating and telescoping. The instability of the medical history. *Arch Intern Med* 2002; **162**: 981–4.
- Jones R, Britten N, Culpepper L, *et al. Oxford Textbook of Primary Medical Care*. Oxford: Oxford University Press, 2003.
- McWhinney IR. *A Textbook of Family Medicine*. Oxford: Oxford University Press, 1997.
- Redelmeier DA, Tu JV, Schull MJ, *et al.* Problems for clinical judgement: 2. Obtaining a reliable past medical history. *CMAJ* 2001; **164**: 809–13.

TEXT REFERENCES

1. Heikkinen M, Pikkarainen P, Eskelinen M, *et al*. GPs' ability to diagnose dyspepsia based only on physical examination and patient history. *Scand J Prim Health Care* 2000; **18**: 99–104.

2. Deyo RA, Diehl AK. Cancer as a cause of back pain: frequency, clinical presentation and diagnostic strategies. *J Gen Intern Med* 1988; **3**: 230–8.

3. Zwietering PJ, Knottnerus JA, Rinkens PELM, *et al*. Arrhythmias in general practice: diagnostic value of patient characteristics, medical history and symptoms. *Family Practice* 1998; **15**: 343–53.

4. Summerton N, Rigby AS, Mann S, *et al*. The general practitioner–patient consultation pattern as a tool for cancer diagnosis in general practice. *Brit J Gen Pract* 2003; **53**: 50–2.

5. Crockett AW. Patterns of consultation and parasuicide. *BMJ* 1987; **295**: 476–8.

6. Van Der Voort JH, Edwards AG, Roberts R, *et al*. Unexplained extra visits to general practitioners before the diagnosis of first urinary tract infection: a case-control study. *Arch Dis Child* 2002; **87**: 530–2.

7. Melbye H, Straume B, Assebo U, *et al*. The diagnosis of adult pneumonia in general practice. *Scand J Primary Health Care* 1988; **6**: 111–17.

8. Summerton N, Paes RA. The clinical assessment of patients with large bowel symptoms by general practitioners. *Eur J Gen Pract* 2000; **6**: 43–7.

9. Peat G, Greig J, Wood L. Diagnostic discordance: we cannot agree when to call knee pain 'osteoarthritis'. *Family Practice* 2004; **22**: 96–102.

10. Honkanen K, Honkanen R, Heikkinen L, *et al*. Validity of self-reports of fractures in perimenopausal women. *Am J Epidemiol* 1999; **150**: 511–16.

11. Rauscher GH, O'Malley MS, Earp JA. How consistently do women report lifetime mammograms at successive interviews? *Am J Prev Med* 2002; **22**: 8–14.

12. Wells JE, Horwood LJ. How accurate is recall of key symptoms of depression? *Psych Med* 2004; **34**: 1001–11.

13. Prior AJ, Darke-Lee AB. Auditing the reliability of recall of patients for minor surgical procedures. *Clin Otol and All Sciences* 1991; **16**: 373–5.

14. Kehoe R, Wu SY, Leske MC, *et al*. Comparing self-reported and physician-reported medical history. *Am J Epidemiol* 1994; **139**: 813–18.

15. Bergmann MM, Calle EE, Mervis CA, *et al*. Validity of self-reported cancers in a prospective cohort study in comparison with data from state cancer registries. *Am J Epidemiol* 1998; **147**: 556–62.

16. Paganini-Hill A, Chao A. Accuracy of recall of hip fracture, heart attack, and cancer: a comparison of postal survey data and medical records. *Am J Epidemiol* 1993; **138**: 101–6.

17. Cochrane AL, Chapman PJ. Observers' errors in taking medical histories. *Lancet* 1951; **1**: 1007–9.

18. Lipworth L, Fryzek JP, Fored CM, *et al*. Comparison of surrogate with self-respondents regarding medical history and prior medication use. *Int J Epidemiol* 2001; **30**: 303–8.

19. Thorogood M, Vessey M. The reliability of surrogate information about oral contraceptive use, smoking, height and weight collected from men about their wives. *Contraception* 1989; **39**: 401–8.

20. Robbins JM, Wolfson CM, Bergman H, *et al.* Agreement between older subjects and proxy informants on history of surgery and childbirth. *J Am Ger Soc* 2000; **48**: 975–9.

21. Malet L, Llorca PM, Boussiron D, *et al.* General practitioners and alcohol use disorders. *Alcoholism* 2003; **27**: 61–6.

22. Ashworth M, Gerada C. ABC of mental health: Addiction and dependence – II: Alcohol. *BMJ* 1997; **315**: 358–60.

23. Aertgeerts B, Buntinx F, Ansoms S, *et al.* Screening properties of questionnaires and laboratory tests for the detection of alcohol abuse or dependence in a general population. *Brit J Gen Pract* 2001; **51**: 206–17.

24. Summerton N, Garrood P. The family history in family practice: a questionnaire study. *Family Practice* 1997; **14**: 285–8.

25. Love RR, Evans AM, Josten DM. The accuracy of patient reports of a family history of cancer. *J Chronic Dis* 1985; **38**: 289–93.

26. Napier JA, Metzner H, Johnson BC. Limitations of morbidity and mortality data obtained from family histories – a report from the Tecumseh Community Health Study. *Am J Public Health* 1972; **62**: 30–5.

27. Kerber RA, Slattery ML. Comparison of self-reported and database-linked family history of cancer in a case-control study. *Am J Epidemiol* 1997; **146**: 244–8.

28. Theis B, Boyd N, Lockwood G, *et al.* Accuracy of family cancer history in breast cancer patients. *Eur J Can Prev* 1994; **3**: 321–7.

29. Floderus B, Barlow L, Mack TM. Recall bias in subjective reports of familial cancer. *Epidemiology* 1990; **1**: 318–21.

30. Douglas FS, O'Dair LC, Robinson M, *et al.* The accuracy of diagnoses as reported in families with cancer: a retrospective study. *J Med Genet* 1999; **36**: 309–12.

31. Aitken J, Bain C, Ward M, *et al.* How accurate is self-reported family history of colorectal cancer? *Am J Epidemiol* 1995; **141**: 863–71.

32. Kee F, Collins BJ. How prevalent is cancer family syndrome? *Gut* 1991; **32**: 509–12.

33. Glanz K, Grove J, Le Marchand L, *et al.* Underreporting of family history of colon cancer: correlates and implications. *Cancer Epidemiol Biomarkers Prev* 1999; **8**: 635–9.

34. Winter PR, Wiesner GL, Finnegan J, *et al.* Notification of a family history of breast cancer: issues of privacy and confidentiality. *Am J Med Genet* 1996; **66**: 1–6.

35. Parent ME, Ghadirian P, Lacroix A, *et al.* Accuracy of reports of familial breast cancer in a case-control series. *Epidemiology* 1995; **6**: 184–6.

36. Schreiber CP, Hutchinson S, Webster CJ, *et al.* Prevalence of migraine in patients with a history of self-reported or physician-diagnosed 'sinus' headache. *Arch Intern Med* 2004; **164**: 1769–72.

37. Headache Study Group of the University of Western Ontario. Predictors of outcome in headache patients presenting to family physicians. A one year prospective study. *Headache* 1986; **26**: 285–91.

38. Smetana GW. The diagnostic value of historical features in primary headache syndromes. *Arch Intern Med* 2000; **160**: 2729–37.

CHAPTER 6

Clinical examination

INTRODUCTION

Having identified and assessed a patient's symptoms, extracted and evaluated other relevant information from the medical history, the next step is to examine the patient.

By writing a separate chapter on the clinical examination I am following the traditional approach but it is important to emphasise that, in reality, there is a much closer integration of the patient's symptoms, their past medical history and the clinical examination. The history-taking conversation will often continue during the course of the clinical examination and some sensitive questions may be more easily asked at this time, possibly prompted by a physical finding.

The iatrotropic problem itself might, perhaps, be a physical finding such as a swelling, a lump or a skin lesion rather than a specific symptom. The patient may even proffer a specific diagnostic concern such as shingles or impetigo. Interestingly, it seems that the patient's subjective report of fever might actually be a more accurate indicator (LR+ = 4.9) of a measured temperature greater than 38°C than the clinician's impression from palpating the patient's forehead (LR+ = 2.5).

As in the case of symptoms, some physical findings may simply represent normal variation and in these circumstances it is necessary to understand the patient's underlying concerns, e.g. the adolescent boy with breast development who is worried that he is undergoing a sex change or is developing cancer. It is also important to be careful about 'regression to the mean' in relation to physical findings that exhibit biological variability and this is one of the arguments in favour of making a number of blood pressure measurements before labelling a patient as hypertensive. As in the case of symptoms and the past medical history, relatives and friends of the patient may also report abnormal physical findings such as a raised temperature or cyanosis.

APPLYING EVIDENCE

One of the greatest difficulties that I have to face as a clinical generalist is deciding which physical findings exhibit (or do not exhibit) a satisfactory level of reliability and validity in my hands and amongst the patients I am likely to encounter on a daily basis. Textbooks about the clinical examination are overflowing with information about eponymous signs, a lot of which seem confusing and obscure. Many are poorly defined and, for those that are described in relation to a number of levels (e.g. some, few, many crackles) the problems are further magnified.

Rather than attempting to separate the wheat from the chaff, it seems that many clinicians have simply ditched the clinical examination. However, there is evidence that, when carefully conducted and focused, it can still provide a wealth of useful discriminant information. Recently I listened to the chest of a patient who had just attended a specialist chest clinic but did not seem as well as usual. He was pyrexial and I was somewhat surprised to be able to detect an obvious pleural rub that had not been noted at the clinic. For a fleeting moment I thought my ausculatory skills must have surpassed those of my specialist colleagues until the patient spluttered 'they don't listen to your chest any longer at the hospital now that they have all 'em scanners'. I sent him on his way with some antibiotics and arranged to see him again a couple of days later.

Predictive validity

The medical history produces a post-history probability that can be adjusted further by the likelihood ratios arising from the clinical examination to produce a new (post-examination) probability of disease. However, it is important to re-emphasise that the post-examination probability is intimately dependent on the post-history probability.

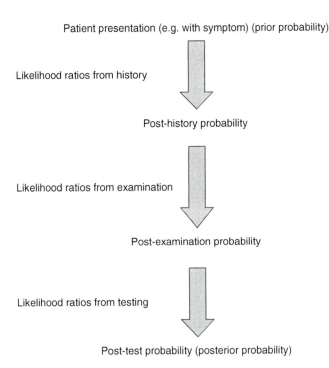

Patient presentation (e.g. with symptom) (prior probability)

Likelihood ratios from history

Post-history probability

Likelihood ratios from examination

Post-examination probability

Likelihood ratios from testing

Post-test probability (posterior probability)

The equations of likelihood ratios in the context of the clinical examination are listed in the Glossary on page 191. Physical findings with positive likelihood ratios greater than 1 increase the probability of disease; the greater the positive likelihood ratio the more compelling the argument for disease. Conversely, physical signs that have positive likelihood ratios between 1 and 0 decrease the probability of disease; the closer the likelihood ratio to zero, the more convincing the finding argues against disease. For example, a palpable gall bladder in a patient with jaundice (Courvoisier's sign) is *in favour* of extrahepatic obstruction of the biliary system (LR+ 26.0) but *against* hepatocellular disorders (LR+ 0.04).

Negative likelihood ratios with values closest to 0 argue the most *against* disease when that clinical finding is absent. For example, in a simple test for hearing impairment the clinician whispers a combination of three letters or numbers while standing about 2 feet behind the patient and then asks them to repeat the sequence. If the patient answers correctly, hearing is considered normal. However, if the individual misidentifies any of the three items, the doctor repeats different triplets twice more. If at least half of the items in the three triplets are incorrect the test is classified as abnormal. This test has particularly good discriminant properties as it indicates significant hearing loss when positive (LR+ = 6.0) but virtually excludes important hearing loss when negative (LR− = 0.03).[1]

A negative likelihood ratio with a value greater than 1 is a little tricky to understand as it assigns some positive diagnostic value to the absence of a finding. One such example is the absence of back pain (LR− = 2.0) in relation to the diagnosis of acute cholecystitis.

As more likelihood ratios are enlisted to seek to cross one of the decision-making thresholds referred to in Chapter 3, care must be taken not to ignore interactions between them. Not all clinical findings are independent and a careful judgement often needs to be made about the wisdom of simply joining together likelihood ratios. For example, although it may be quite legitimate to multiply the positive likelihood ratios for diminished breath sounds (LR+ = 2.3) and an elevated temperature (LR+ = 2.0) in relation to a putative diagnosis of pneumonia, it would not seem so reasonable to link together the positive likelihood ratios for shifting dullness (LR+ = 2.3) and a positive fluid wave (LR+ = 5.0) for the detection of ascites. In less clear-cut situations, where the possibility of interactions between physical findings is more uncertain, it may be best to focus exclusively on the single best clinical examination item and its likelihood ratio. An alternative approach is to use 'clinical information clusters' that have been selected using logistic regression techniques or likelihood ratios that have been statistically adjusted. In a study in a Canadian hospital setting it was demonstrated that both these approaches improved the diagnosis of airflow limitation in comparison with simply multiplying likelihood ratios.[2] Moreover there was little to choose between picking the best sign (auscultated wheezing) or developing information triplets (smoking duration, reported wheezing, auscultated wheezing).

One of the particular difficulties faced by primary care practitioners seeking to make a diagnosis is that, no matter how rigorous their history taking, the post-history probability will still generally be lower than amongst similar patients attending specialist clinics as a direct result of the lower disease prevalence (prior [pre-history] probability) within the community setting. Statistically derived information clusters can be particularly valuable in seeking to address this problem by both enhancing the magnitude of likelihood ratios and accounting for interactions between clinical signs and symptoms (*see also* page 35).

In a prospective study of 201 patients with possible sinusitis attending 35 general practitioners in Norway, a cross-sectional comparison was made of items of clinical information against CT scan results (the diagnostic reference standard) in order to identify positive likelihood ratios (*see* Table 6.1).[3]

Thus, in this situation, simply multiplying the individual likelihood ratios would have overestimated their combined discriminatory power by 15%. One other interesting finding from this study was that many other traditional signs such as sinus tenderness did not produce significant likelihood ratios.

Reliability

Reliability and the use of kappa have been discussed in previous chapters and often seem to be under-emphasised compared to the predictive validity and the use of likelihood ratios. However, no matter how good the diagnostic validity, a finding from the clinical examination is virtually useless if different observers vary in their ability to elicit the finding. Moreover, although a sign may show excellent agreement between specialists (e.g. heart sounds and cardiologists), for diagnosis in primary care what really matters is the consistency between generalists.

My clinical examination may be unreliable for a number of reasons. On a home visit I might discover that my otoscope batteries are running out or that the only earpiece I have in my bag is too narrow. In examining a patient's chest I might not be using my stethoscope optimally or my percussion strokes may be too forceful. Sometimes I can be less attentive or become distracted; or as a result of my training I may be better at eliciting some signs (and worse at others) than my colleagues. I might also exhibit bias; physical signs are always much more obvious to me once

TABLE 6.1 Diagnosis of sinus infection in general practice

Clinical information	Positive likelihood ratio
Double sickening (two phases in the illness history)	2.1
Purulent rhinorrhoea	1.5
Purulent secretion in cavum nasi	5.5
ESR > 10 mm/h	1.7
All four items present	25.2

someone else (or an ultrasound scan in the case of an enlarged spleen or liver) has identified them! However, some matters are beyond my control such as biological variation or some signs are just too vague. For example, deciding whether a peripheral pulse is absent or present demonstrates moderate to almost perfect agreement between observers (kappa 0.52–0.92) but assessing whether a pulse is 'normal' or 'diminished' is so subjective that is highly unreliable (kappa 0.01–0.15).

Reliability might be improved by training, possibly using a number of aids such as models, videos, CDs and even simulated and 'standardised' patients. However, it may be that some physical signs are simply too precise in relation to the type of decisions we are seeking to make as primary care clinicians. In patients presenting with a unilateral red eye the challenge for me lies in distinguishing relatively benign conditions (e.g. conjunctivitis) from serious pathology (e.g. iritis or keratitis). Recent research in a primary care setting has revealed that a pen-light test during which a pocket flashlight (3 volts) is shone directly on to an eye for 2 seconds from a distance of 15 cm may be particularly helpful. A positive result, defined as the patient reporting 'additional discomfort', was shown to have a positive likelihood ratio of 4.2 and a negative likelihood ratio of 0.2 for serious eye pathology in general practice.[4]

Finally, when examining a patient it is clear that some features such as a rash, blood pressure, temperature or pulse rate can be objectively measured whereas others such as lung sounds are more open to subjective interpretation. However, it would be incorrect to assume that such objective measurements should always be trusted. In checking a patient's blood pressure, errors may arise from, for example, the use of the wrong sized cuff (the bladder should encircle at least 80% of the upper arm) or the incorrect positioning of the arm (the arm should be at heart level). Blood pressure should also be measured in both arms, as there may be differences of as large as 10 mmHg between arms.[5]

THE PRELIMINARY ASSESSMENT

Nowadays in many family/general practices patients are summoned into the consulting room by means of electronic boards, loudspeakers or receptionists. In other more traditional set ups the doctor walks into the waiting room and invites the patient in. If we are going to practise primary care diagnostics I would argue that it is important to appreciate that the 'clinical examination' commences from the moment we clap eyes on the patient. If we simply sit immobile in our consulting rooms we might easily miss the difficulty a patient with polymyalgia rheumatica can have rising from the waiting room chair. Observation of the patient's gait as they walk down the corridor can provide important information on neurological or musculoskeletal problems. In one study of the diagnosis of Parkinson's disease, a shuffling gait provided a positive likelihood ratio of 3.3, difficulty rising from a chair 1.9, whereas tremor only added 1.4.[6] Emotions can also affect walking; some depressed patients have a characteristic gait, marked by a shorter stride and weaker push-off with the heel when compared with non-depressed individuals.[7]

It is also important to appreciate that even the waiting room is a carefully controlled environment and home visits can still provide a valuable insight into a patient's problems. Nailing down a stair carpet and changing a light bulb certainly helped to address the problem of recurrent bruising in one of my elderly patients.

PATIENT OBSERVATION

Once the patient arrives in the consulting room, and during the course of the subsequent clinical interview, careful observation ought to continue. Intriguingly, a recent study of patients in one UK general practice has shown that right-handed people with anxiety and depression were more likely to choose to sit on the left of the doctor in a consultation (and *vice versa*) when given the choice.[8] The author suggests that orienting behaviour may be disturbed in states of anxiety and depression (although in one surgery where I worked I suspect that a rather dubious looking stain on one of the chairs in the consulting room may also have contributed to the patient's seat selection!).

Personally I have worried about my use of the computer during the consultation ever since an elderly women remarked about a colleague, 'I'm not going to see Doctor X anymore; he never looks at me; he just stares at the television.' Primary care diagnostics must be about making the most appropriate use of technology at every stage of the diagnostic processing pathway and to keep as much attention as possible directly focused on the patient.

A wealth of information may be gained by careful observation of the patient long before we reach for our medical bag. This can incorporate straightforward clinical findings such as anaemia/jaundice to providing an insight into the patient's health behaviour, emotional state or general wellbeing. Even a glance at the dentition may help; a tooth count of less than 20 has a positive likelihood ratio of 3.4 for osteoporosis.[9]

I am confident that I can smell a smoker (or a passive smoker) at 2 yards. Others emphasise the use of nicotine stained fingers and nails to assess both current and previous smoking status. Half-stained nails indicate recent smoking cessation (a fingernail grows at a rate of 0.1 mm per day) and if the nails are also clubbed (LR+ = 3.9 for lung cancer) this might indicate a possible reason why the patient may have altered their behaviour. In a prospective study of patients attending a general medical outpatient clinic half of the current cigarette smokers who had smoked for 10 years or more could be identified by their facial features alone, i.e. gaunt look, leathery skin, excessive skin wrinkling, and both grey and unduly ruddy skin hues.[10]

When I commenced in single-handed practice in Yorkshire I had to undergo the usual round of visits from some of the local elderly ladies just to 'check on the new doctor'. In retrospect, what was most notable about these visits was that the health of my visitors both then, and over the subsequent 5 years, seemed to bear an intriguingly close relationship to their use of make-up. Interestingly, other work has demonstrated a 'lipstick sign' amongst ladies in hospital who begin to re-apply their lipstick when they are recovering from an illness.[11] Recently (and rather against my own preferences) I agreed to manage an 80-year-old woman at home with quite a significant chest infection. I think the sign that was of most significance in demonstrating her recovery was to arrive at her house one day and to find her having her hair permed by the mobile hairdresser.

Listening and observing is self-evidently good clinical practice but as indicated in the previous chapters there is also a requirement to assess the validity and the reliability of the information obtained. It is also necessary to make a judgement as to whether any research producing likelihood ratios or kappa values to describe such clinical information is applicable to the primary care-based clinical encounter.

Although we are taught that jaundice becomes easy to diagnose clinically once the serum bilirubin exceeds 3 mg/dL, it seems that only 70% of primary care physicians can actually detect jaundice at this threshold. Furthermore, despite the finding that the recognition of jaundice may demonstrate substantial agreement between different doctors (kappa = 0.65), it is noteworthy that 7% of doctors will still miss jaundice if the bilirubin level exceeds 15 mg/dL.

The most compelling clinical findings arguing for anaemia are conjunctival rim pallor (LR+ = 16.7) and palmar crease pallor (LR+ = 7.9) whereas my favourite physical sign (nail bed pallor) only achieves a paltry positive likelihood ratio of 1.7. Importantly no physical sign convincingly argues against the diagnosis of anaemia (i.e. no likelihood ratio is less than 0.5). In terms of reliability, conjunctival rim pallor also demonstrates a kappa value of 0.65 (substantial agreement between observers) compared to a kappa of 0.27 for my nail bed pallor (only slight agreement between observers). Perhaps the time has come to adjust this element of my clinical examination!

THE PURPOSES OF THE CLINICAL EXAMINATION

Echoing the clinical interview, examining the patient is not simply about diagnosis – it also has therapeutic and legal elements. It often seems to me that if a patient perceives that they have had a 'thorough' (and courteous) examination they are often much more likely to be comfortable with my clinical judgement. In contrast, if I rigidly adhere to those elements of the clinical examination that I consider have sufficient validity or reliability I sometimes find it more difficult to reassure the patient.

Primary care diagnostics is about trying to see the world through the patient's eyes and then to move on to assess the discriminant value of the clinical information obtained. However, before we lay hands on a patient it is important to be quite clear about objectives. For example, if I listen to a patient's chest – is it to assist me in the diagnosis? (in which case, am I confident about reliability and validity?) or is it to help to reassure the patient? (in which case, am I being honest with the patient?)

or is it for 'doctor-centred' reasons, such as defensive medical practice or to appear competent in the eyes of my professional colleagues and/or superiors? On my part I know that I certainly use the clinical examination to give me thinking time in the context of a continuing conversation with the patient. However, such multi-tasking can have its downsides; more than once I have had to re-check a blood pressure as my mind was focused more on the diagnostic possibilities than the diastolic!

I would argue that it is particularly important to be clear about both the purpose and the predictive validity/reliability if the patient is going to be subjected to something particularly unpleasant or embarrassing such as a rectal or a vaginal examination. In 1990 Hennigan *et al.* criticised general practitioners for their reluctance to perform rectal examinations.[12] However, although there is some evidence that the rectal examination may have a role in the assessment of men with urinary problems, there is nothing to recommend the procedure as part of the routine gynaecological assessment in women.[13] Moreover a case-control study showed no benefit of routine digital rectal examination in reducing mortality from cancer of the distal rectum.[14] In addition to these findings, a survey of internal medicine residents in Minneapolis revealed that most doctors had received little formal instruction in undertaking a rectal examination and ensuring patient comfort.[15] Patients were frequently uncertain why the examination had been performed and lacked any understanding of the results of the examination.

CLINICAL PROBLEMS

In the remainder of this chapter I shall discuss some selected clinical problems that have caused me difficulties in order to illustrate the assistance provided by the clinical examination (and research judged applicable to the primary care setting).

Acute/sub-acute abdominal pain

I often seem to encounter younger patients with acute abdominal pain or discomfort and the initial differential diagnosis in such patients is broad, incorporating gastrointestinal conditions, biliary/hepatic problems, urological conditions, gynaecological/obstetric pathology, muscular pain, extra-abdominal conditions (e.g. basal pneumonia) and a number of rare haematological and biochemical abnormalities. Data on the diagnoses in over 10 000 patients with acute abdominal pain reveal that inflammation of the appendix and gall bladder represent the majority of acute abdominal problems referred to surgical departments. In addition, many conditions such as abdominal muscle wall pain, gastro-enteritis and urinary tract infections are managed exclusively within primary care.

Is the pain likely to be related to the urinary tract?

In a woman with lower abdominal pain and/or flank pain certain symptoms and signs may assist in the diagnosis of urinary tract infections (*see* Table 6.2).

TABLE 6.2 Likelihood ratios for urinary tract infections in women

Clinical feature	Positive likelihood ratio	Negative likelihood ratio
Dysuria	1.5	0.5
Frequency	1.8	0.6
Haematuria	2.0	0.9
Fever	1.6	0.9
Vaginal discharge	0.3	3.1
Vaginal irritation	0.2	2.7
Back pain	1.6	0.8
Self-diagnosis	4.0	0.1
Vaginal discharge on examination	0.7	1.1
Costovertebral angle tenderness on examination	1.7	0.9
Dipstick analysis (positive for leucocyte esterase or nitrite)	4.2	0.3

Thus a urinary tract infection is more likely if a woman has dysuria, frequency, haematuria, back pain and costovertebral angle tenderness. The individual positive likelihood ratios with the greatest magnitude are provided by the dipstick analysis and also by the patient's own view about the likely diagnosis (the absence of these findings is also useful to exclude a urinary tract infection in view of the low negative likelihood ratios). The *absence* of vaginal discharge or irritation also confers significant negative likelihood ratios, thereby further increasing the likelihood of a urinary tract infection. Furthermore, the symptom combination 'presence of dysuria and frequency but absence of vaginal discharge and irritation' provides an overall likelihood ratio of 24.6.[16]

Aside from urinary tract infections, renal colic due to ureterolithiasis also needs to be considered. Information derived from a study of 1333 patients with acute abdominal pain revealed that loin tenderness (LR+ = 27.7, LR– = 0.9), renal angle tenderness (LR+ = 3.6, LR– = 0.2), and, especially, microscopic haematuria (LR+ = 73.1, LR– = 0.3) were the key factors to take into account.

Could it be appendicitis?

Many of my patients attend with a concern that their abdominal pain might be appendicitis. It is always very satisfying to get this diagnosis correct but it can be quite tricky and textbooks are full of (sometimes contradictory) advice. Table 6.3 shows the likelihood ratios that have been identified.[17]

It is important to appreciate that some of these signs (i.e. rigidity, guarding, rebound tenderness and cough tenderness) are also general signs for peritonitis/peritoneal irritation. However, finding a patient with pain and tenderness in the

TABLE 6.3 Likelihood ratios for the diagnosis of appendicitis

Clinical feature	Positive likelihood ratio	Negative likelihood ratio
Right lower quadrant pain	7.3–8.5	0.3
Migration of pain	3.2	0.5
Pain before vomiting	2.8	na*
Fever	1.8	0.5
Rigidity (involuntary muscle contraction)	4.0	0.8
Guarding (voluntary muscle contraction)	2.2	0.5
Right lower quadrant tenderness	7.3	0.1
McBurney's point tenderness	3.4	0.4
Rebound tenderness	2.0	0.5
Positive cough test	2.4	0.3
Rovsing's sign (pressure over the patient's left quadrant causing pain in the right lower quadrant)	2.5	0.7

* Not applicable.

right iliac fossa, especially if they have McBurney's point tenderness, a positive cough test and a positive Rovsing's sign argues strongly in favour of appendicitis. One caveat is that some of the signs listed above that appear to have reasonable likelihood ratios exhibit poor inter-observer reliability. The kappa value for guarding is 0.36 (slight agreement), for rebound tenderness 0.25 (slight agreement) and for rigidity is only 0.14 (poor agreement).

Could it be cholecystitis?

The majority of patients encountered in primary care settings with upper abdominal pain are subsequently found to have a relatively benign cause for the pain but acute cholecystitis still warrants consideration (*see* Table 6.4).[18]

Murphy's sign refers to pain and arrested inspiration occurring when an examiner's fingers are hooked underneath the right costal margin during deep inspiration. A positive Murphy's sign together with the presence of right upper quadrant tenderness/pain, fever and vomiting argue for cholecystitis. The presence of back tenderness argues against the diagnosis possibly because it is found more commonly in alternative diagnoses such as renal disease or pancreatitis. There is little information on the reproducibility of Murphy's sign but, in general, there is less confidence in its value for patients over the age of 60 years.

Clearly this is not an exhaustive list but it serves to illustrate and highlight some of the available evidence. Gastric problems (e.g. peptic ulceration), pancreatitis and a range of other possibilities also may need considering along similar lines. More generally, some workers have sought to assess the accuracy of the examination of

TABLE 6.4 Likelihood ratios for acute cholecystitis

Clinical feature	Positive likelihood ratio	Negative likelihood ratio
Right upper quadrant pain	1.5	0.7
Right upper quadrant tenderness	1.6	0.4
Fever	1.5	0.9
Vomiting	1.5	0.6
Nausea	1.0	0.6
Rebound tenderness	1.0	1.0
Murphy's sign	2.8	0.5
Back tenderness	0.4	2.0

the abdominal organs as well as the detection of ascites. Unfortunately, finding an enlarged spleen or an enlarged liver by percussion or palpation is neither particularly valid or reliable.[19,20] Even if a clinician palpates a liver edge extending below the costal margin this does not necessarily indicate hepatomegaly (LR+ = 1.7) and to assess the liver span by percussion is very unreliable (kappa = 0.11, poor agreement). A palpable spleen does argue in favour of splenomegaly (LR+ = 9.6) and the level of inter-observer agreement of the finding ranges from a kappa of 0.56 to 0.70 (moderate to substantial agreement) but, unfortunately, many enlarged spleens are impalpable.

General abdominal distension is not a particularly reliable sign (kappa = 0.35, slight agreement) but some features in the history and the examination can assist in the identification of ascites (*see* Table 6.5).[21]

TABLE 6.5 Likelihood ratios for ascites

Clinical feature	Positive likelihood ratio	Negative likelihood ratio
Increased girth	4.2	0.2
Recent weight gain	3.2	0.4
Hepatitis	3.2	0.8
Ankle swelling	2.8	0.1
Heart failure	2.0	0.7
Alcoholism	1.4	0.7
History of cancer	0.9	1.0
Bulging flanks	2.0	0.3
Flank dullness	2.0	0.3
Shifting dullness	2.7	0.3
Fluid wave	6.0	0.4
Peripheral oedema	3.8	0.2

Thus the most useful signs for making a diagnosis of ascites are a positive fluid wave, shifting dullness and peripheral oedema. To rule out ascites a negative history of ankle swelling, no increase in abdominal girth and an inability to demonstrate bulging flanks, flank dullness, shifting dullness or peripheral oedema are most helpful.

A poorly child

As a primary care physician I obviously encounter a lot of children in my day-today practice. I have discussed meningitis earlier, but two particular problems I often seem to have to face are detailed below.

Does the child have otitis media?

Acute otitis media is responsible for at least 30 million patient visits per annum in the US (and at a cost exceeding 5 billion dollars). Furthermore, considerable energy has been devoted to examining the most effective treatment and in discussing the role of antibiotics. However, from my perspective as a primary care clinician, recognition rather that treatment is what I find most perplexing. I also suspect that I am not alone, and it has been suggested that, in general, primary care physicians are unsure about the diagnosis at least 40% of the time. Such uncertainty may result in increased use of antibiotics, antibiotic resistance and unnecessary referrals, and can also lead to other causes of fever or illness being misdiagnosed as acute otitis media. In a group of children with acute otitis media, 90% had fever, ear pain, crying and irritability (*see* Table 6.6) but 72% of children unwell but without acute otitis media complained of exactly the same symptoms.[22]

Thus in a child with ear pain and/or reported ear rubbing the most useful findings in the ear are a cloudy or bright red and bulging ear drum. Drum redness also

TABLE 6.6 Likelihood ratios for acute otitis media

Clinical feature	Positive likelihood ratio	Negative likelihood ratio
Ear pain	3.0	0.6
Ear rubbing	3.3	0.7
Fever	0.8	1.2
Cough	0.9	1.2
Rhinitis	1.3	0.6
Excessive crying	1.8	0.7
Cloudy drum	11	na*
Very red drum	2.6	na
Bulging drum	20	na
Poorly mobile drum (pneumatic otoscopy)	8.4	na

* Not applicable.

TABLE 6.7 Likelihood ratios for 5% dehydration in children

Clinical feature	Positive likelihood ratio	Negative likelihood ratio
Prolonged capillary re-fill	4.1	0.6
Abnormal skin turgor	2.5	0.7
Abnormal respiratory pattern	2.0	0.8
Sunken eyes	1.7	0.5
Dry mucous membranes	1.7	0.4
Cool extremity	1.5	0.9
Absent tears	2.3	0.5
Sunken fontanelle	0.9	1.1

exhibits less inter-observer variability (kappa = 0.40, slight agreement) than bulging (kappa = 0.16, poor agreement). Interestingly, in a recent study of primary care physicians in Scandinavia it seems that most base their diagnoses on the symptoms and the colour of the tympanic membrane, whereas their specialist ENT colleagues paid more attention to the movement and the position of the tympanic membrane.[23]

Is the child dehydrated?

Dehydration is often a concern in children who have had vomiting, diarrhoea or a poor oral intake. Although I have been unable to identify any studies from primary care, 13 studies have been undertaken in hospital and emergency department settings.[24] The likelihood ratios for these are shown in Table 6.7.

The problem with many of these signs is that they are very non-specific and exhibit considerable inter-observer variability. The range of kappa values is shown in Table 6.8.

TABLE 6.8 Kappa ranges for symptoms used to assess 5% dehydration in children

Clinical feature	Range of kappa values
Prolonged capillary re-fill	0.01–0.65
Abnormal skin turgor	0.36–0.55
Abnormal respiratory pattern	−0.04–0.40
Sunken eyes	0.06–0.59
Dry mucous membranes	0.28–0.59
Cool extremity	na*
Absent tears	0.12–0.75
Sunken fontanelle	0.10–0.27

* Not applicable.

Thus from this evidence it seems that sunken eyes, a sunken fontanelle and dry mucous membranes offer little help in making a positive diagnosis of 5% dehydration due to the low likelihood ratios and the range of kappa values (from poor to moderate agreement). Dehydration is less likely in the absence of dry mucous membranes as this exhibits the lowest negative likelihood ratio and also has a more acceptable range of kappa values than many of the other physical signs.

However, in assessing children it is always important not to ignore the information elicited from the parents: certainly parental report of normal urine output (e.g. assessed by the number of wet nappies during a defined time period) has been reported as having negative likelihood ratios of 0.16 and 0.27. Personally I also assess if the child looks unwell or if the parents seem particularly concerned. This re-emphasises that, although likelihood ratios may offer considerable assistance, they need to be considered in conjunction with clinical experience and other patient-derived information, which may not be quite so easy to quantify.

Capillary re-fill time and skin turgor have the highest positive likelihood ratios but asking around colleagues it does seem that some of the inter-observer variation and unreliability may reflect differences in the way these signs are elicited. Steiner *et al.* advocate the standardisation of these features (*see* Box 6.1).[24]

Box 6.1 Standardisation of clinical assessment for dehydration in children

How to assess capillary re-fill time	The room should be well lit and warm.
	• The arm should be held at the level of the heart and pressure should be gradually increased on the palmar surface of one of the patient's fingertips until the capillary bed blanches.
	• The pressure is then released immediately and, in non-dehydrated children, the colour should return in less than 2 seconds.
How to assess skin turgor	• The examiner should use the thumb and index finger to pinch a small skin fold on the lateral abdominal wall at the level of the umbilicus. The fold is then promptly released and the time taken to return to normal is classified (somewhat unsatisfactorily!) as immediate, slightly delayed or prolonged.

An older person with headaches

Temporal arteritis is a particular concern in older patients who present to me with headaches. Although the prevalence is estimated to be only 0.15% for patients over the age of 50, timely diagnosis and treatment with high-dose steroids can prevent visual loss. Moreover, although most primary care clinicians are well aware that ESR has a place in the diagnosis of the condition, insufficient emphasis is often given to the information obtained directly from the patient via the history or the clinical examination.[25]

There is a range of reported symptoms and signs for temporal arteritis and the positive and negative likelihood ratios for these are shown in Table 6.9.[26]

The headache of temporal arteritis is often non-specific in character and it seems that a temporal location only confers a positive likelihood ratio of 1.5 and a tender scalp only 1.6. Jaw claudication is pain in the proximal jaw near the temporomandibular joint that develops after a brief period of chewing (especially for food requiring a lot of mastication such as tough meat) and provides a higher positive

TABLE 6.9 Likelihood ratios for temporal arteritis

Clinical feature	Positive likelihood ratio	Negative likelihood ratio
Anorexia	1.2	0.9
Weight loss	1.3	0.9
Arthralgia	1.1	1.0
Diplopia	3.4	0.9
Fatigue	1.2	0.9
Fever	1.2	0.9
Temporal headache	1.5	0.8
Jaw claudication	4.2	0.7
Myalgia	0.9	1.1
Polymyalgia rheumatica	1.0	1.0
Unilateral visual loss	0.9	1.2
Any visual symptom	1.1	1.0
Vertigo	0.7	1.1
Scalp tenderness	1.6	0.9
Beaded temporal artery	4.6	0.9
Prominent or enlarged temporal artery	4.3	0.7
Tender temporal artery	2.6	0.8
Absent temporal artery pulse	2.7	0.7
Any temporal artery abnormality	2.0	0.5

TABLE 6.10 Range of ESR in patients referred for temporal artery biopsy

Range of ESR (mm/hr)	Positive likelihood ratio
< 21	0.0
21–40	0.5
41–60	0.3
61–80	1.4
81–100	3.2
> 100	2.3

likelihood ratio of 4.2. However, no information is available on the reproducibility of this symptom and it must also be distinguished from disorders of the temporomandibular joint where the pain commences immediately on mastication. The presence of diplopia also substantially increases the likelihood of disease (LR+ 3.4). However, it is important to note that the negative likelihood ratios of jaw claudication and diplopia are only 0.7 and 0.9 respectively, indicating that their *absence* is much less helpful in arguing *against* the diagnosis of temporal arteritis.

Upon examination, a number of abnormalities of the temporal artery (i.e. tenderness, beading, prominence and absent pulsation) increases the probability of temporal arteritis. Conversely, the absence of any temporal artery abnormality is the examination feature with the lowest negative likelihood ratio (i.e. the absence of temporal artery abnormalities argues against temporal arteritis).

One further issue that needs to be considered in relation to the diagnosis of temporal arteritis is the *additional value* of the ESR. When the ESR is raised the interpretation should really depend on the clinician's pre-test (post-history/examination) estimate of the probability of arteritis. Table 6.10 shows ESR findings in patients referred for temporal artery biopsy who, presumably, will have a high pre-test probability of temporal arteritis.

Applying Bayes' Theorem (*see* Chapters 3 and 5) it can be calculated that when the pre-test probability is low, a normal ESR reduces the probability of disease to less than 1%. Once the ESR rises above 61 mm/hr the posterior (post-test) probability would be increased.

If the pre-test probability is as high as 70% (i.e. jaw claudication, diplopia and temporal artery findings) then, when the ESR is between 41 and 60 mm/hr, the probability of temporal arteritis would be *reduced* to 41%. It may be difficult to decide what to do with the patient in such a situation but I would contend that the risk to the vision is such that we are still above at least one of the decision-making thresholds referred to in Chapter 3 and further action (treatment or investigation) should be considered. The key point is that the information extracted from the patient *should not* be ignored in favour of the ESR result.

A person with chest problems

I might examine a patient's chest for a number of reasons but, most commonly, I am interested in detecting evidence of infection or heart failure. In determining whether an adult has a community-acquired pneumonia a number of clinical features have been suggested (*see* Table 6.11).[27]

Although some individual findings such as a raised respiratory rate, an elevated temperature, dullness to percussion and bronchial breath sounds provide substantial positive likelihood ratios, clusters of findings are more powerful. A combination of a temperature of greater than 37.8°C, a heart rate more than 100 beats per minute, crackles, diminished breath sounds in a patient without asthma provides a positive likelihood ratio of 8.2, while the absence of this combination produces a negative likelihood ratio of 0.3.

In relation to predicting left ventricular dysfunction in patients aged 70–84 living in the community, basal crackles in the chest confer a positive likelihood ratio of 2.4.[28] However, this needs to be considered in relation to a history of breathlessness (LR+ = 5.4), a past history of myocardial infarction (LR+ = 4.3) or angina (LR+ = 3.3). Also many elderly patients have co-existing chronic obstructive pulmonary disease and, in such individuals, the combination of a history of ischaemic heart disease, a body mass index > 30, a laterally displaced apex beat, a heart rate greater than 90 beats per minute, and a raised BNP level confers a positive likelihood ratio of 5.6 (negative likelihood ratio 0.7).

TABLE 6.11 Likelihood ratios for pneumonia diagnosis in adults

Clinical feature	Positive likelihood ratio	Negative likelihood ratio
Cough	1.8	0.3
Dyspnoea	1.4	0.7
Sputum production	1.3	0.6
Fever	2.1	0.7
Chills	1.6	0.9
Night sweats	1.7	0.8
Myalgias	1.3	0.6
Respiratory rate > 25 breaths/minute	3.4	0.8
Heart rate > 120 beats/minute	1.9	0.9
Temp > 37.8°C	4.4	0.8
Dullness to percussion	4.3	0.8
Decreased breath sounds	2.5	0.6
Crackles	2.7	0.9
Bronchial breath sounds	3.5	0.9

TABLE 6.12 Kappa values for chest signs

Clinical feature	Kappa value
Reduced percussion note	0.52
Wheezes	0.51
Pleural rub	0.51
Reduced breath sounds	0.43
Crackles	0.41
Bronchial breathing	0.32
Tachypnoea	0.25

Unfortunately, one of the particular difficulties of the chest examination is the unreliability of some of the physical findings (*see* Table 6.12).[29]

Others have found that dichotomous variables such as wheezes, crackles and rubs are more reliably detected than graded variables such as dullness and breath sound intensity.[30] In children it seems that there is better agreement about signs that can be observed such as the use of accessory muscles, colour and attentiveness.[31] The reliability of assessing the respiratory rate (the absence of which is the best individual finding for ruling out pneumonia in children) can be improved by counting for 60 seconds.

In a study of the diagnosis of pneumonia in general practices in Norway (at an earlier stage in the illness), Melbye and colleagues emphasised that, whatever the findings of the chest examination they should not be used to overrule a typical history of dyspnoea, chest pain and fever in the diagnosis of pneumonia in younger adults.[32] They further emphasise the importance of the information derived from vital signs such as temperature, respiratory rate and pulse rate.

Finally, one other condition that always needs to be considered in the differential diagnosis of a patient presenting with pleuritic chest pain, haemoptysis or dyspnoea is pulmonary embolism. Chest examination may reveal crackles, a pleural rub and, in up to 11% of patients with pulmonary emboli, chest wall tenderness and in 7% an elevated temperature. A history of cancer (LR+ = 4.1), calf pain or swelling (LR+ = 2.6) and tachycardia (LR+ = 2.5) support a diagnosis of embolism but it is important to be aware that the only finding that argues against an embolism is a heart rate less than 90 beats per minute (LR+ = 0.3). Since a misdiagnosis is potentially fatal, there should always be a low threshold for further investigation of such patients.[33]

GENERAL REFERENCES
- Jones R, Britten N, Culpepper L, *et al. Oxford Textbook of Primary Medical Care.* Oxford: Oxford University Press, 2003.
- McGee S. *Evidence-Based Physical Diagnosis.* Philadelphia: WB Saunders, 2001.

TEXT REFERENCES

1. Bagai A, Thavendiranathan P, Detsky AS. Does this patient have hearing impairment? *JAMA* 2006; **295**: 416–28.

2. Holleman DR, Simel DL. Quantitative assessments from the clinical examination. How should clinicians integrate the numerous results? *J Gen Intern Med* 1997; **12**: 165–71.

3. Lindboek M, Hjortdahl P, Johnsen ULH. Use of symptoms, signs and blood tests to diagnose acute sinus infections in primary care: comparison with computed tomography. *Fam Med* 1996; **28**: 183–8.

4. Yaphe J, Pandher KS. The predictive value of the penlight test for photophobia for serious eye pathology in general practice. *Family Practice* 2003; **20**: 425–7.

5. Williams B, Poulter NR, Brown MJ, *et al.* Guidelines for the management of hypertension. *J Human Hypertens* 2004; **18**: 139–85.

6. Rao G, Fisch L, Srinivasan S, *et al.* Does this patient have Parkinson's disease? *JAMA* 2003; **289**: 347–53.

7. Sloman L, Berridge M, Homatidis S, *et al.* Gait patterns of depressed patients and normal subjects. *Am J Psych* 1982; **139**: 94–7.

8. Luck P. Does the presence of psychological distress in patients influence their choice of sitting position in face-to-face consultation with the GP? *Laterality* 2006; **11**: 90–100.

9. Green AD, Colon-Emeric CS, Bastian L, *et al.* Does this woman have osteoporosis? *JAMA* 2004; **292**: 2890–900.

10. Model D. Smoker's face: an underrated sign? *BMJ* 1985; **291**: 1760–2.

11. Kaplan AI, Sabin S. The lipstick sign. *Ann Intern Med* 1981; **94**: 137.

12. Hennigan TW, Franks PJ, Hocken DB, *et al.* Rectal examination in general practice. *BMJ* 1990; **301**: 478–80.

13. Campbell KA, Shaughnessy AF. Diagnostic utility of the digital rectal examination as part of the routine pelvic examination. *J Fam Pract* 1998; **46**: 165–7.

14. Herrinton LJ, Selby JV, Friedman GD, *et al.* Case-control study of digital-rectal screening in relation to mortality from cancer of the distal rectum. *Am J Epidemiol* 1995; **142**: 961–4.

15. Wilt TJ, Cutler AF. Physician performance and patient perceptions during the rectal examination. *J Gen Intern Med* 1991; **6**: 514–17.

16. Bent S, Nallamothu BK, Simel DL. Does this woman have an acute uncomplicated urinary tract infection? *JAMA* 2002; **287**: 2701–10.

17. Wagner JM, McKinney WP, Carpenter JL. Does this patient have appendicitis? *JAMA* 1996; **276**: 1589–94.

18. Trowbridge RL, Rutkowski NK, Shojania KG. Does this patient have acute cholecystitis? *JAMA* 2003; **289**: 80–6.

19. Grover SA, Barkun AN, Sackett DL. The rational clinical examination. Does this patient have splenomegaly? *JAMA* 1993; **270**: 2218–21.

20. Naylor CD. The rational clinical examination. Physical examination of the liver. *JAMA* 1994; **271**: 1859–65.

21. Williams JW, Simel DL. The rational clinical examination. Does this patient have ascites? *JAMA* 1992; **267**: 2645–8.

22. Rothman R, Owens T, Simel DL. Does this child have acute otitis media? *JAMA* 2003; **290**: 1633–40.

23. Blomgren K, Pitkaranta A. Is it possible to diagnose acute otitis media accurately in primary care? *Family Practice* 2003; **20**: 524–7.

24. Steiner MJ, DeWalt DA, Byerley JS. Is this child dehydrated? *JAMA* 2004; **291**: 2746–54.

25. Sox HC. *Common Diagnostic Tests: use and interpretation.* Philadelphia: American College of Physicians, 1990.

26. Smetana GW, Shmerling RH. Does this patient have temporal arteritis? *JAMA* 2002; **287**: 92–101.

27. Metlay JP, Kapoor WN, Fine MJ. Does this patient have community-acquired pneumonia? *JAMA* 1997; **278**: 1440–5.

28. Morgan S, Smith H, Simpson I, *et al.* Prevalence and clinical characteristics of left ventricular dysfunction among elderly patients in general practice setting: cross sectional survey. *BMJ* 1999; **318**: 368–72.

29. Spiteri MA, Cook DG, Clarke SW. Reliability of eliciting physical signs in examination of the chest. *Lancet* 1988; **1**: 873–5.

30. Mulrow CD, Dolmatch BL, Delong ER, *et al.* Observer variability in the pulmonary examination. *J Gen Intern Med* 1986; **1**: 364–7.

31. Margolis P, Gadomski A. Does this infant have pneumonia? *JAMA* 1998; **279**: 308–13.

32. Melbye H, Straume B, Assebo U, *et al.* The diagnosis of adult pneumonia in general practice. *Scand J Prim Health Care* 1988; **6**: 111–17.

33. Chunilal SD, Eikelboom JW, Attia J. Does this patient have a pulmonary embolism? *JAMA* 2003; **290**: 2849–58.

CHAPTER 7

Diagnostic testing

INTRODUCTION

A couple of years ago I admitted one of my charming elderly female patients into the local community hospital. The problem was an infected and swollen foot that had defied my best therapeutic endeavours and I wondered if the time had come for intravenous antibiotics. Following her subsequent discharge I visited her again at home and, although the foot looked remarkably similar, the patient was considerably perkier.

She recounted that my hospital colleagues, having been unable to insert a drip for antibiotics, had become concerned that she might actually have a deep-vein thrombosis. Unfortunately, the appropriate diagnostic machinery was located 20 miles away so ambulance transport was arranged. She told me that she had had a lovely day out travelling the scenic route along the coast. When she returned to the hospital clutching her normal investigation results and a stick of seaside rock her discharge was arranged without further ado.

Although I am always delighted to encounter a contented patient, I was a little bewildered about the need for the investigation (and the 40-mile round trip). If there had been a deep-vein thrombosis my patient would, presumably, have been treated with the anticoagulant, warfarin. There was only one problem with this: the patient had been on a maximum dose of warfarin for the previous 10 years!

Diagnostic processing can involve a number of investigations ranging from simple urine dipsticks to more elaborate technologies such as radiology, endoscopy, physiological and pathological testing. However, primary care diagnostics is not simply about assimilating masses of information from as many of these tests as possible in order to detect or to exclude a disorder, it is also about considering the risks and the benefits of any investigation from the perspective of the patient. Furthermore, it is necessary to place the patient in context and to assess the impact of testing on the individual's family and the limited healthcare budget.

Many problems associated with the use of investigations could be avoided if we considered more carefully how the result of the test would influence the patient's clinical course. Some inappropriate testing is undertaken to exclude unlikely diseases (in which case many of the positives may simply be false positives), others to confirm diagnoses that are already established or for which there may be no treatment (or any required treatment change). As discussed in Chapter 2, a significant number of investigations are performed for 'non-clinical' reasons, such as defensive medical practice.

Biochemical tests such as rheumatoid factor or cancer antigen 125 (CA-125) are often used inappropriately by some primary care physicians. CA-125 is a high molecular weight glycoprotein that is expressed by 80% of epithelial ovarian cancers. In view of the insidious nature of ovarian cancer with no specific symptoms it has been suggested that this test may be of some diagnostic assistance. Unfortunately, only about 50% of patients with stage 1 disease have elevated CA-125 levels (risk of false negatives). Furthermore, in a recent review of 799 patients who had undergone the test in a hospital setting (where patients will, presumably, be more 'selected' to undergo the test than in primary care) it was shown to have a very high false-positive rate often due to certain benign conditions such as fibroids, endometriosis and early pregnancy. The authors concluded that the inappropriate usage of CA-125 has led to results that are useless to the clinician, have significant cost implications and add to patient anxiety and clinical uncertainty.[1]

Rheumatoid factor may also be used inappropriately by some primary care clinicians without sufficient consideration of the findings obtained from an assessment of the patient's symptoms, their past medical history or from the clinical examination. In a Canadian study of patients referred to rheumatologists by primary care physicians, prior requests for rheumatoid factor (and any positive results) were examined in relation to patients' final rheumatological diagnoses (*see* Table 7.1).[2]

The results indicate that most tests were negative and were often ordered in patients without any pre-test evidence for connective tissue diseases. In such circumstances the impact of the test result on the post-test probability of disease would be tiny. The authors suggested that more effective and efficient use of rheumatoid factor could be achieved by emphasising that symptoms such as fatigue and diffuse musculoskeletal pain are not indicative of connective tissue diseases in the absence of other features such as joint swelling, a typical rash or organ involvement.

In Chapter 3 I discussed the importance of being clear about the clinical question as clinical information can be used for a range of different purposes. For example, B-type natriuretic peptide (BNP) might be used for prognostic prediction, risk stratification, therapeutic monitoring or for screening in addition to the diagnosis of heart failure. However, two further issues need to be re-emphasised in relation to diagnostic testing.

1   What particular condition(s) is being sought (or excluded)?
2   What is the most appropriate test (or combination of tests) to use?

TABLE 7.1 Measurement of rheumatoid factor and rheumatological diagnoses

Rheumatological diagnosis	Proportion in which rheumatoid factor requested (%)	Proportion of requests that showed a positive result (%)
Rheumatoid arthritis	56	72
Systemic lupus erythematosus	50	25
Spondyloarthropathies	27	0
Other connective tissue diseases	26	12
Spinal pain syndromes	14	12
Osteoarthritis	18	22
Localised osteoarticular rheumatism	24	10
Other soft-tissue rheumatism	18	10
Crystal arthropathies	29	29
Other rheumatic diseases	11	100
Diseases primarily from other systems	14	25
Syndromes not diagnosed	54	20
No diseases	80	0

Nowadays it is all-to-easy to send patients off for a battery of investigations without a clear view about the likely diagnostic possibilities. It is a good exercise in primary care diagnostics to both write down (and also share with the patient) the most probable diagnoses before reaching for the pathology or radiology request form. It is also much simpler to discuss the likelihood of anxiety or depression accounting for the symptoms if these issues have been raised with the patient *before* any more complex testing commences.

It is important to appreciate that, for many investigations, 'normal' is defined in relation to the overall distribution of the results obtained from a number of individuals. For most biochemical tests this 'reference range' is designed to accommodate 95% of the results for patients without disease. Thus 1 in 20 of 'abnormal' results may not be truly abnormal but simply outside this defined range. Moreover, as a patient is subjected to more such tests, the greater are the chances of an 'abnormal' result. It can be calculated that, after performing 14 tests the odds of a 'false abnormal' result will have risen from one in 20 to one in two. It could be considered that a 'normal' patient is simply one who has been insufficiently investigated!

So far in this book I have worked along the diagnostic pathway prospectively from symptoms to medical history and on to the clinical examination. However, when arranging investigations it is often more helpful to think

backwards and consider what would be the next step if the result of the test turned out to be:
- positive
- negative
- equivocal.

Recently I was consulted by a 4-year-old child (together with his parents and grand-parents) who had typically enlarged, but resolving, jugulo-digastric lymph nodes. The problem was that he had previously been seen by a 'hospital-centred' locum doctor who had arranged a white cell count. The child's sore throat was improv-ing, as expected from the natural history of such conditions, but I was now faced with anxious parents/grandparents, a crying child and report from the laboratory stating that the sample had been unsatisfactory and needed repeating. Particularly with children, there is a requirement to think very carefully about the need for often-distressing blood tests. Personally, if I am concerned, a second opinion from an experienced paediatrician is my preferred first-line 'investigation'. In the case of adults, I have encountered at least two patients who have undergone 'normal' liver biopsies (a procedure not without risk) as a consequence of an ill-considered tick on a biochemistry request form.

Wald suggests that the following issues should always be considered prior to arranging any diagnostic test.[3]
1   What disorder is being tested for?
2   What is the natural history of the disorder (i.e. is it a self-limiting or a trivial condition)?
3   How common is the disorder (i.e. is there a high chance of a false-positive result)?
4   What are the predictive validity and reliability of the investigation?
5   How will the result of the investigation influence clinical action?
6   Are the risks of the investigation *and* any subsequent investigations, procedures and therapy known and judged to be acceptable in the light of the needs of the patient?

When a number of alternative tests are available a careful balance often needs to be struck between their discriminant properties (predictive validity and reliability), the risk of adverse effects and the costs. Table 7.2 weighs up these three issues in relation to the diagnosis of urinary tract stones.[4]

TABLE 7.2 Diagnostic tests for urinary tract stones

Test	Discriminant properties	Risk of adverse effects	Relative cost
Urine dipstick	+	minimal	$
Ultrasound	++	minimal	$$
IVP	+++	5–0%	$$$$
Helical CT	++++	minimal	$$$

All investigations must also be carefully considered in relation to the information already obtained from the symptoms, the past medical history and the clinical examination that will have produced a post-examination probability of disease.

Patient presentation (e.g. with symptom) (prior probability)

Likelihood ratios from history

Post-history probability

Likelihood ratios from examination

Post-examination probability

Likelihood ratios from testing

Post-test probability (posterior probability)

Thus in some situations diagnostic testing will add little to the information that has already been obtained. In other words the test/action thresholds will already have been crossed and the post-history/post-examination probabilities may be such that a decision can now be reached without the requirement for further testing.

Irritable bowel syndrome

The recognition of irritable bowel syndrome is a particular challenge as the diagnosis is based on the occurrence of typical symptoms and the exclusion of a range of other conditions such as inflammatory bowel disease, gastrointestinal infections and colorectal cancer. The Manning and Rome criteria for the diagnosis of irritable bowel are listed in Table 7.3.[5]

From the patient's perspective the concern is that they may be subjected to increasingly invasive and somewhat risky investigations. For example, colonoscopy has a serious adverse event rate of between 0.4% and 1.2% with an overall mortality of about 0.01%. Furthermore, it was estimated that the excess medical cost for diagnosing irritable bowel syndrome in the US (in 1992) was $8 billion.

Suleiman and Sonnenberg adopted a Bayesian approach to examine the diagnostic processing pathway for patients with possible irritable bowel syndrome.[6] Based on a prior probability of 5%, they estimated that a post-test probability of 80%

TABLE 7.3 Criteria for irritable bowel syndrome.

Manning criteria	Rome I criteria	Rome II criteria
Abdominal distension Pain relief with bowel movement More frequent stools with pain Looser stools with pain Mucus per rectum Feeling of incomplete evacuation	> 3 months of continuous or recurrent symptoms: • abdominal pain relieved with defecation and/or associated with a change in stool consistency. *Plus* two or more of the following on at least 25% of days: – altered stool frequency (> 3 per day or < 3 per week) – altered stool form (lumpy/hard or loose/watery) – altered stool passage (straining, urgency, or feeling of incomplete evacuation) – passage of mucus – bloating or feeling of abdominal distension	> 12 weeks of continuous or recurrent symptoms: • abdominal pain or discomfort. *Plus* at least two of the following: – relieved with defecation and/or – associated with change in frequency of stool and/or – associated with change in form (appearance) of stool

could be achieved by relying solely on relatively inexpensive and non-invasive tests (i.e. the history, the clinical examination, faecal occult blood testing, a full blood count, a measurement of thyroid stimulating hormone, liver and kidney function tests, serum electrolytes, albumin, coagulation and a stool sample [for culture, ova/ parasites and giardia faecal antigen] together with hydrogen breath testing) and without the need for sigmoidoscopy or colonoscopy. As a result of this work they suggest a carefully staged approach to the diagnosis of irritable bowel syndrome and that the endoscopic procedures should be scheduled at the end of the diagnostic pathway. However, they added the important caveat that colonoscopy/sigmoidoscopy is still indicated in patients in whom ruling out serious organic disease is required after the initial processing (e.g. aged over 50 and alarm symptoms such as rectal bleeding or unexplained weight loss).

Parkinson's disease

Shortly after I had first started in general practice I was called to see a man who lived just around the corner from the surgery. On entering the house I took one look at the patient and made an immediate diagnosis of Parkinson's disease. He was shuffling around the room with an expressionless face, all his movements were slow and he had an obvious tremor. However, I was a little perplexed when the patient's wife looked disappointed rather than elated by my rapid assessment. 'The last four GPs who visited also though it was Parkinson's disease ... and you are wrong too', she said, passing me a recent letter from a neurologist.

As discussed in Chapter 3 primary care diagnostics is not only about emphasising the importance of the information obtained directly from the patient and using it more rationally, it is also about assessing the validity and the reliability of such data. In some circumstances the likelihood ratios might be too small, the research study in which they were developed of dubious quality and/or there may be concerns about inconsistencies between doctors in the way information is abstracted or interpreted. Consequently it is always necessary to appreciate that, in some situations, seeking a specialist opinion or undertaking further investigations may be the only sensible option.

Whereas a diagnosis of Parkinson's disease might be straightforward in some patients it can be very challenging in others. Misdiagnoses occur most commonly in patients with essential tremor, drug-induced parkinsonism and vascular parkinsonism. Seventy-five per cent of patients with Parkinson's disease complain of a tremor that is said to occur at rest. According to the textbooks it is also coarse, unilateral, 'pill-rolling' and has a frequency of 3–5 Hz. Unfortunately, in many patients the tremor is less typical and can also be intermittent or seen only when the patient is walking. Even for a neurologist, distinguishing Parkinson's disease from other parkinsonian syndromes such as progressive supranuclear palsy or multisystem atrophy can be quite tricky. Clinicopathological studies based on brain bank material from the UK and Canada have shown that clinicians diagnose the disease incorrectly in about 25% of patients.[7]

Mistaking Parkinson's disease for other conditions can lead to inappropriate and ineffective treatment. While a patient with essential tremor may benefit from a beta-blocker, this treatment will have no impact on the tremor of Parkinson's disease. Incorrect treatment based on misdiagnosis also delays the use of dopaminergic medications, which can decrease the severity of symptoms and disability. From the patient's perspective delayed diagnosis can generate considerable anxiety as only once the condition has been recognised and treated can patients plan for their future and make sensible social and domestic adjustments. Treating patients without Parkinson's disease with anti-parkinsonian medications can also be harmful. Dyskinesias and hallucinations can occur in over 20% of patients given levodopa. There is also evidence that levodopa causes damage to dopamine neurones in non-Parkinsonian patients.

According to a recent review the positive likelihood ratio of new-onset tremor for the diagnosis of Parkinson's disease is 1.3 and, even combined with rigidity and bradykinesia, only makes 2.2.[8] Even a good treatment response to levodopa provides a surprisingly tiny positive likelihood ratio of 1.4. Thus, taking the prior probability of Parkinson's disease in a patient over the age of 65 to be 1%, it seems unlikely that the history and the examination could push this up to more than 20%. To compound matters further there are major concerns about the reliability of the clinical assessment in relation to such signs as cogwheel or lead-pipe rigidity, the assessment of bradykinesia or the glabella tap. Some symptoms and signs such as micrographia, trouble turning over in bed or difficulty in opening jars have been suggested to have greater reliability and validity but the studies supporting these findings are of consistently low quality.

Thus in relation to the rational diagnosis of Parkinson's disease there is certainly a place for new diagnostic technologies. Possible tools include olfactory testing using 'Sniffin Sticks' and single photon emission computed tomography (SPECT) imaging. DaTSCAN is the radiopharmaceutical agent ioflupane 123 which, when injected intravenously, becomes attached to the dopamine transporters (DAT protein) in the pre-synaptic nigrostriatal nerve endings. SPECT imaging can then be used to quantify any changes in the patient's dopamine transporters, an early diagnostic marker for Parkinson's disease. Particularly important from the patient's perspective, there is no need to withdraw anti-parkinsonian treatment before or during the test. DaTSCAN has been shown to exhibit a sensitivity of 97% and a specificity of 100% in distinguishing essential tremor from Parkinsonian syndromes. It has also been successfully used to differentiate Parkinson's disease from the parkinsonian condition multisystem atrophy.[7]

In the reminder of the chapter I focus on three particular areas of concern in relation to the use of investigations by primary care clinicians: near-patient testing, open-access radiology services and approaches to encouraging the more rational use of investigations by primary care clinicians.

NEAR-PATIENT LABORATORY TESTING

The current drive to deliver more services within primary care settings is re-focusing attention on near-patient testing. Such testing is defined as the performance of any pathological investigation outside a laboratory where the result is available without the sample being sent to a laboratory for analysis.

Near-patient testing includes urinalysis, biochemistry and pregnancy testing together with more recent innovations such as D-dimer testing for deep-vein thrombosis, assessment of myocardial damage using troponin, microbial antigen assays, e.g. for *H. Pylori* and *Chlamydia*, and the estimation of inflammatory markers such as C-reactive protein (CRP). Near-patient testing also allows international normalised ratio (INR) monitoring in patients on warfarin and diabetic monitoring using serial glycated haemoglobin (HbA1c) measurements. With the on-going rapid developments in genetics and micro-technology the future possibilities are legion.

Some are attracted to near-patient testing by the potential for cost savings, enhanced speed and patient satisfaction. Near-patient tests are often promoted as being cheaper by virtue of, for example, reduced sample transport costs. However, there is a requirement to balance this against the increased capital costs with possible duplication of testing and the reduced efficiency where activity volumes are low. There is also a need to consider the running costs from reagents, quality control procedures, maintenance and training. Many hospital laboratories also continue to express concerns about the dubious quality assurance processes and the training deficiencies associated with many of the existing near-patient testing systems being used within primary care settings with consequent adverse impacts on patient wellbeing.

It is imperative that the attraction of the technology does not distract our attention from the requirement for a continuing focus on the importance of the other information derived directly from the patient in the context of the history and the clinical examination. It is well recognised that the presence of a new service stimulates activity and there is a particular need to be confident that any investigation (whether it is near-patient or laboratory based) is only used after a careful consideration of risks and benefits. As for any investigation, the ultimate value of a near-patient test in primary care must be assessed by its impact on patient care.

The diagnosis of deep-vein thrombosis

The clinical diagnosis of deep-vein thrombosis (DVT) is a particular problem in primary care. In a recent meta-analysis of individual clinical features, only a history of malignancy (LR+ 2.7), previous DVT (LR+ 2.3), recent immobilisation (LR+ 2.0), difference in calf diameter (LR+ 1.8) and recent surgery (LR+ 1.8) were useful in providing some evidence in favour of the diagnosis.[9] However, none of these likelihood ratios is particularly dramatic and there is also a concern about the burgeoning use of expensive and potentially invasive radiology being used to exclude the diagnosis.

D-dimer is a degradation product of a cross-linked fibrin blood clot. Levels are raised in the presence of a DVT in addition to a range of other situations/conditions such as recent major surgery, haemorrhage, trauma, pregnancy, cancer or acute arterial thrombosis. As discussed in Chapter 3 negative likelihood ratios with values closest to zero argue the most *against* disease when a test result is negative. The negative likelihood ratio for DVT when the D-dimer test is negative is, on average across a number of studies, 0.20 and this could significantly reduce the post-examination/pre-test probability.

In clinical practice, scoring systems are often used to assess a patient's pre-test probability of DVT. The Well's scoring system shown in Table 7.4 was developed and validated using data from 593 out-patient referrals and exhibits excellent test-retest reliability. Patients are given a score from −2 to 9 and the probability of DVT is said to be 'high' if the score is above 3, 'moderate' if it is 1 or 2 and 'low' if it is 0 or less.[10]

A moderately sensitive D-dimer test providing a negative result could shift a pretest probability for DVT of 5% to a new post-test probability of 1.0% perhaps making further investigation or referral unnecessary. However, a patient with a high pre-test probability of 53% would still have a probability of 18% after testing negative and, in this situation the D-dimer result may have less impact on the clinical outcome. Clearly the purpose of undertaking any D-dimer test should always

TABLE 7.4 Clinical model for assessment of deep-vein thrombosis (Well's score)

Clinical variable	Score
Active cancer (treatment on-going or within previous 6 months or palliative)	1
Paralysis, paresis, or recent plaster immobilisation of the lower extremities	1
Localised tenderness along the distribution of the deep venous system	1
Recently bedridden for 3 days or more, or major surgery within the previous 12 weeks requiring general or regional anaesthesia	1
Entire leg swollen	1
Calf swelling at least 3 cm larger than on the asymptomatic leg (measured 10 cm below the tibial tuberosity)	1
Pitting oedema confined to the symptomatic leg	1
Collateral superficial veins (non-varicose)	1
Previously documented DVT	1
Alternative diagnosis as least as likely as DVT	−2

be carefully considered in relation to the pre-test probability (e.g. from the Well's score) and there is a need to guard against allowing the result to provide unwarranted reassurance in patients at high risk.[11]

More recently it has also been suggested that the Well's rule, alone or in combination with D-dimer testing, does not guarantee accurate estimates of risk in primary care patients in whom DVT is suspected.[12] The problem of applying clinical decision rules to different settings was discussed in Chapter 3 and it is now suggested that consideration also be given to an alternative rule developed within primary care[13]; *see* Table 7.5.

TABLE 7.5 New clinical model for assessment of DVT

Variable	Points
Male	1
Use of hormonal contraceptives	1
Active cancer in past 6 months	1
Surgery in previous month	1
Absence of leg trauma	1
Distention of collateral leg veins	1
Difference in calf circumference ≥ 3 cm[†]	2
Abnormal D-dimer assay result	6

[†]Calf circumference was measured 10 cm below the tibial tubercle.

This new rule combines clinical information with D-dimer testing and reduces the need for onward referral for suspected DVT by 50% with a low risk of subsequent venous thromboembolic events.

Acquiring diagnostic information rapidly

Many of the advocates of near-patient testing highlight the ability to obtain results rapidly with improved patient care and enhanced patient satisfaction. Compared to traditional laboratory testing, collection time, transport time, analysis time and reporting time are all reduced. However, in a review of near-patient testing in an accident and emergency department, although faster changes in treatment were achieved in 7% of patients, such changes had no significant impact on patient outcomes.[14]

As primary care clinicians we are all aware of the importance of admitting a patient with a suspected myocardial infarction into hospital as soon as possible. We also need to be familiar with the possibility of false-negative rates of any investigation; in a proportion of patients with a myocardial infarction the ECG will be quite normal and the cardiac enzymes may not be raised. I am therefore always at a loss to understand why some colleagues choose to delay admission of a patient with chest pain until they have undertaken a troponin test. Desktop analysis for troponin has a sensitivity for a final diagnosis of myocardial infarction of 33% within 2 hours of the onset of pain and 86% after 8 hours.[15] If the clinical suspicion is sufficient to warrant undertaking such a near-patient test then surely it would seem more logical to simply admit the patient directly on to the coronary care unit. In this situation the near-patient test appears to represent an unwarranted and somewhat risky delay.

At the other end of the spectrum is the patient who has an unexplained symptom. In these circumstances an immediate result may not allow time for the symptom to evolve (when the patient returns for review) or for the patient and their doctor to reflect further on the likely cause of the symptom. As emphasised in Chapter 4, many symptoms are 'unexplained' and over-investigation of such symptoms might cause significant harm. In our enthusiasm for near-patient testing we must not neglect time as a diagnostic and therapeutic tool.

In between these two extremes there are situations where immediate testing may be of possible benefit. Examples include an ESR in an elderly patient with headaches, glucose and ketone testing in a patient with diabetes or INR testing in a patient on warfarin. Antibiotic prescribing may also be targeted more effectively through the use of near-patient CRP measurement.[16]

Quality assurance

In common with any information being used for diagnostic decision making in primary care there is a requirement to be confident about the reliability and the validity of near-patient testing. Unfortunately, the majority of studies of near-patient tests have been conducted outside primary care settings and primary care clinicians need to know the nature of the study population if they are going to give meaning to the likelihood ratios. There is often a tendency to recruit cohorts of either healthy, self-selected volunteers such as medical students or less well populations from out-patient clinics. This is important, as clinical information may only be positive in extensive/advanced disease or in less well patients but negative in localised disease or in situations where there are significant co-morbidities. Near-patient testing machine manufacturers might only provide performance data for their equipment under ideal conditions and they should be encouraged to undertake and publicise the data derived from primary care populations.

Reliability of results is normally assured by internal and external quality control procedures. Internal quality control generally involves the use of 'standard reagents' in order to assess how consistent the near-patient test results are on a day-to-day basis. In external quality control schemes near-patient testing sites are sent unknown samples to analyse and then return their results to a co-ordinating laboratory. These results can be used to help to assess the near-patient testing site's performance in relation to others.

There has been a lot of concern about the lack of effective quality assurance in primary care near-patient testing. This can have significant impacts on patients: over an 8-year period in the US glucose meter inaccuracies were blamed for 24 deaths and 986 injuries according to federal data.[17] However, it would be wrong to assume that laboratory readings are universally reliable as other/different sources of error may occur in the laboratory. Samples might be mixed up or incorrectly stored, and there can be inaccuracies in transcribing results and during the transmission of the results back to the primary care clinician.

It has been argued that conventional external quality control procedures are tedious, time-consuming and difficult to undertake in primary care. An alternative suggested approach is to consider the near-patient testing site as a satellite of an accredited laboratory. Quality assurance could then be undertaken by sending random, duplicate samples to the laboratory for comparison with the near-patient testing result. However, there is a need to appreciate that simply submitting second samples of extreme results to the laboratory is open to errors arising from the phenomenon of 'regression to the mean'. As a result of this the near-patient tester may gain the impression (falsely) that their machine always reads higher than the laboratory result and makes inappropriate adjustments to his or her care. It is also important to be confident that it is reasonable to compare finger prick near-patient testing using capillary blood against a laboratory result derived from a venous sample. Errors may also arise from the interpretation of a result either by laboratory staff or by primary care clinicians. Much laboratory advice is often confounded by a lack of awareness about key pieces of clinical information such as the patient's current medication or physiological conditions, e.g. pregnancy. In contrast, a primary care physician sitting with a patient and a near-patient testing machine ought to be particularly well placed to consider the test result in the context of the patient. But few of us have trained as chemical pathologists or haematologists and we may lack the requisite skills to read results correctly and interpret the findings appropriately. More sophisticated near-patient testing is probably best combined with some form of computerised decision support to provide advice on the significance of results and their implications for future management. Most examples at present relate to anticoagulation control but other systems are being developed.

OPEN-ACCESS DIAGNOSTIC SERVICES

Many primary care physicians now enjoy open access to a range of more complex investigations such as radiology, ultrasound, echocardiography, endoscopy and MRI. However, with such enhanced access comes the additional responsibility to ensure the effective, efficient and appropriate use of such investigations (*see* Table 7.6). It is particularly important to guard against being seduced by the technology and to forget the patient. It is also necessary to appreciate that such high technology tests suffer from deficiencies in relation to predictive validity and reliability in exactly the same way as does the history or the clinical examination.

Recently I decided to undergo training in flexible sigmoidoscopy. Generally I consider myself to be quite practical, but I was nearly defeated by this task: I got lost, twisted, stuck and frequently blinded by residual stool in the bowel. I also had to keep being reminded that the primary purpose of the investigation was not simply to reach the splenic flexure (and then get out again!) without causing too much distress to the patient, but rather to spot any likely pathology. As a primary care clinician I learnt two broader lessons from this experience: first that I had insufficient understanding about what more complex investigations really entailed (especially in terms of patient discomfort and distress) and second that (at least in some operators' hands) the findings may not be as believable as I once thought.

Table 7.7 shows the level of inter-observer agreement in relation to some of the most common investigations.

Some investigations such as ECGs, spirometry or audiology may be undertaken either in a primary care setting or as an 'open-access' service. In such circumstances

TABLE 7.6 Some possible adverse effects of open-access diagnostics

- the potential for a 'cascade' effect with mildly abnormal results generating further tests
- adverse effects arising from diagnostic delay (due to inappropriate or inefficient testing)
- risk of physical and psychological harm to patients (both from the test and from any subsequent action or inaction)
- increased demand for testing and less appropriate referrals with a consequent reduction in diagnostic yield
- impact on patient/health service finances

TABLE 7.7 Kappa values for some common investigations

Investigation	Indication	Kappa value
Chest radiograph	Detection of cardiomegaly	0.48
Chest radiograph	Detection of oedema	0.83
Contrast venography	DVT in leg	0.53
Head CT scan after stroke	Normal or abnormal?	0.60
MRI of spine	Disc: normal or abnormal?	0.59
Calf ultrasound	Calf DVT	0.69
Ultrasound of thyroid	Nodule: yes or no?	0.57–0.66
Endoscopy	Grade of reflux oesophagitis	0.55
Liver biopsy (pathological examination)	Cirrhosis	0.59
Liver biopsy (pathological examination)	Alcoholic liver disease	0.49

where the test involves an element of interpretation it is very important to be 'operator aware'. For example, spirometry interpretation has been shown to exhibit a kappa of 0.31 between chest physicians but only –0.12 between general practitioners in my local area.

Chest radiographs make up a large proportion of the expenditure on diagnostic technology. Worldwide it is estimated that they account for half of all radiological procedures. However, the reasons for taking a chest radiograph can often be somewhat obscure and they have been used variously for screening and for diagnosis. It has also been promoted as a more sensitive method of detecting occult chest disease (especially lung cancer or tuberculosis) than the assessment of symptoms, the medical history or the clinical examination.

In the 1950s/1960s in order to assess the predictive validity of the chest radiograph, 6027 male volunteers aged 45 or older living in Philadelphia were radiologically screened every 6 months for 10 years and questioned about symptoms and smoking habits.[18] They were self-selected volunteers and some were lost to follow-up. The risk of lung cancer according to the clinical features is shown in Table 7.8.

Thus the medical history and symptoms are more powerful clinical predictors of lung cancer than the radiographic findings. However, misinterpretation of the result of a chest radiograph can be a factor in the delayed diagnosis of lung cancer. In a study from Hull, UK, the most common reason for a diagnosis of lung cancer to be missed was a failure of the radiologist reporting the radiograph to recognise the abnormality.[19] In a separate study from Russia agreement between radiologists on the presence or the absence of an abnormality on a chest radiograph was only fair (kappa = 0.38).[20] Intriguingly, even intra-observer agreement (i.e. the same radiologist viewing the same radiograph on different occasions) exhibited only moderate to good reliability (kappa = 0.53–0.63).

TABLE 7.8 Lung cancer risk percentages

Clinical feature	Risk of lung cancer (%)
Lung fields clear on chest X-ray on entry to study and asymptomatic	1.78
Lung fields unclear on chest X-ray on entry to study (i.e. non-specific lung disease)	2.64
Chronic cough	2.98
Hoarseness	3.42
Coughing smokers (i.e. more than one pack/day for 40 years)	8.81

In using the results from chest radiographs there is a need to be aware that false-positive and false-negative results can arise for several reasons. For example, poor exposure, poor patient positioning, patient motion and lack of cooperation may all lead to artefacts and might obscure significant findings on the film. Even with perfect technique, lesions can be hidden by overlying shadows or normal structures may be incorrectly interpreted as pathological findings. In one study half of the patients with haemoptysis had a normal chest radiograph[21] and, as patients with haemoptysis generally warrant referral anyway whatever the result of the chest radiograph, I now generally refer such patients at the same time as ordering the chest radiograph in order to minimise delay.

In a study of patients attending a day hospital the chest radiograph was demonstrated to have most value (in terms of altering patient management) in patients with pre-existing cardio-respiratory symptoms and signs.[22] In patients presenting to primary care physicians with acute cough, the presence of rhinorrhea, a sore throat, a respiratory rate < 25 breaths per minute, a temperature < 100°F and the *absence* of night sweats, myalgia and sputum production there is a minimal risk of pneumonia and it is suggested that a chest radiograph can be avoided.[23]

In terms of heart failure diagnosis, vascular redistribution and cardiomegaly are held up as the best individual radiographic findings to diagnose left ventricular dysfunction.[24] However, the kappa values are only 0.50 and 0.48, respectively, and the positive likelihood ratios are also only 2.0 for vascular redistribution and 2.4 for cardiomegaly. Furthermore, a recent review examining the use of B-type natriuretic peptide (BNP) has demonstrated that, in combination with an ECG, BNP can provide a positive likelihood ratio of 4.5 for the diagnosis of left ventricular systolic dysfunction.[25]

ENHANCING THE APPROPRIATE USE OF INVESTIGATIONS

Nowadays as I gain access to an increasingly wide range of investigations I am becoming concerned that my understanding of the indications for such tests is not as good as it should be, which presents an increased risk of inappropriate use.

Computed tomography (CT) scanning of the abdomen delivers a radiation dose equivalent to 500 chest radiographs or 4.5 years of background radiation. However, a recent study reported the results of such scanning amongst a group of patients presenting to family practitioners in California with non-acute abdominal pain.[26] Unsurprisingly, in the light of the information presented in Chapter 4, the majority of patients (60%) received no firm diagnosis and those that did already had an obvious warning feature derived from their symptoms, the medical history or the clinical examination.

In relation to the assessment of back problems in primary care CT scanning and magnetic resonance imaging seem to have taken the place of lumbar spine radiographs amongst some of my primary care clinical colleagues. However, in a recent systematic review, it was concluded that, in the absence of systemic disease or progressive neurological deficit, imaging is usually not required in patients with acute back pain of less than 6 weeks duration.[27]

There is always the concern that, at this point in the diagnostic processing pathway, the primary care approach can easily be forgotten. Moreover, there is a risk that the earlier steps in the diagnostic pathway (and the pre-test probability) are ignored once the patient reaches the radiology department. Primary care diagnostics must therefore also be about the establishment of a two-way dialogue between primary care clinicians and the testing clinicians. Undoubtedly, as primary care physicians we could provide the radiologist with more helpful information on the following:

- symptoms
- past medical history (i.e. surgery, current medication and illnesses)
- previous imaging history
- current infectious diseases (especially diarrhoea/vomiting and methicillin-resistant *Staphylococcus aureus*)
- last menstrual period and risk of pregnancy
- presence of metallic foreign bodies, aneurysm clips, pacemakers and cochlear implants (especially for patients undergoing MRI)
- what the patient has been told about the most likely diagnosis (and what diagnoses we are attempting to confirm or exclude).

Furthermore, I would suggest that primary care clinicians ordering any specialised investigation should:

- have a reasonable view of the likely diagnostic possibilities and outcomes based on the medical history and the clinical examination
- be aware of the minimum data requirements for effective onward diagnostic processing, including maximising the opportunities for effective feedback and subsequent decision support
- be aware of the most appropriate next step(s) in the diagnostic processing pathway together with the subsequent sequence depending on the outcome of the first investigation
- be equipped to discuss with the patient the risks and benefits of the initial test and any likely subsequent tests, procedures and therapy.

For certain investigations it might even be appropriate to develop 'pre-entry' requirements. This could involve the specification of a minimum data set including features from the medical history, the clinical examination and as a result of simple investigations. The clinician ordering the investigation could also be required to specify the purpose of the request in terms of patient outcome(s). Such a minimum data set would be collected and transmitted to the diagnostic tester (e.g. radiologist) before the patient is permitted to undergo more complex diagnostic processing. The approach should ensure that the additional testing is necessary, appropriate and that any feedback is better able to support clinical decision making.

Several years ago my colleagues and I undertook a project with a radiologist and a group of general practitioners in Yorkshire in order to seek to rationalise requests for lumbar spine radiographs.[28] Using a modified radiology request form we asked a group of general practitioners in Huddersfield to specify the reason for their referral (i.e. to make a diagnosis, to exclude a diagnosis, at the patient's request or for medico-legal reasons). During the 1-year study, and compared to a control group of doctors in the neighbouring community of Halifax, general practitioners in Huddersfield were significantly less likely to request lumbar spine radiographs. In The Netherlands a much bigger study was undertaken at around the same time as our work in order to focus on a much broader range of investigations over a longer time period.[29] For 8 years, 85 general practitioners in the city of Maastricht were provided with regular individualised feedback on their test ordering and the appropriateness of the investigations requested. The advice transmitted back to the participating doctors was based on the best available evidence and incorporated general recommendations such as the avoidance of further testing when the pre-test probability (based on the history and the examination) was already high. The impact on the test requesting over the study period was dramatic (*see* Table 7.9).

Furthermore, over the same period there was a nationwide trend of yearly increases of 7–8% in diagnostic testing within primary care.

TABLE 7.9 Reductions in test requests in Maastricht over eight years.

Investigation	Percentage reduction
Haematology	39
Serology	60
Biochemistry	30
Urine/faeces tests	48
Bacteriology/virology	17
ECG	4
Radiology	0

From the clinician's perspective, there appeared to be a general learning effect on the ordering of *all* diagnostic tests. Furthermore, the study provides an indication of the possible economic value of a patient-centred approach to test ordering. By the end of the 8 years (in 1991) the 85 participating practices had saved money ($2 per patient) even after taking into account the costs of the feedback.[29] Moreover, this saving was achieved without any increase in hospital referrals and other work has also demonstrated that such an approach is not accompanied by adverse health outcomes.[30]

GENERAL REFERENCES

- Jones R, Britten N, Culpepper L, *et al. Oxford Textbook of Primary Medical Care.* Oxford: Oxford University Press, 2003.
- McGee S. *Evidence-Based Physical Diagnosis.* Philadelphia: WB Saunders, 2001.
- Sox HC. *Common Diagnostic Tests: use and interpretation.* Philadelphia: American College of Physicians, 1990.

TEXT REFERENCES

1. Moss EL, Hollingworth J, Reynolds TM. The role of CA-125 in clinical practice. *J Clin Pathol* 2005; **58**: 308–12.
2. Suarez-Almazor ME, Gonzalez-Lopez L, Gamez-Nava JI, *et al.* Utilisation and predictive value of laboratory tests in patients referred to rheumatologists by primary care physicians. *J Rheumatol* 1998; **25**: 1980–5.
3. Wald N. *Rational Use of Investigations in Clinical Practice.* London: Royal College of Physicians, 1990.
4. Lindbloom EJ. What is the best test to diagnose urinary tract stones? *J Fam Pract* 2001; **50**: 657–8.
5. Fass R, Longstreth GF, Pimentel M, *et al.* Evidence- and consensus-based practice guidelines for the diagnosis of irritable bowel syndrome. *Arch Intern Med* 2001; **161**: 2081–8.
6. Suleiman S, Sonnenberg A. Cost-effectiveness of endoscopy in irritable bowel syndrome. *Arch Intern Med* 2001; **161**: 369–75.
7. Tolosa E, Wenning G, Poewe W. The diagnosis of Parkinson's disease. *Lancet Neurol* 2006; **5**: 75–86.
8. Rao G, Fisch L, Srinivasan S, *et al.* Does this patient have Parkinson's disease? *JAMA* 2003; **289**: 347–53.
9. Goodacre S, Sutton AJ, Sampson FC. Meta-analysis: the value of clinical assessment in the diagnosis of deep venous thrombosis. *Ann Intern Med* 2005; **143**: 129–39.
10. Wells PS, Owen C, Doucette S, *et al.* Does this patient have deep vein thrombosis? *JAMA* 2006; **295**: 199–207.
11. Fancher TL, White RH, Kravitz RL. Combined use of rapid D-dimer testing and estimation of clinical probability in the diagnosis of deep vein thrombosis: systematic review. *BMJ* 2004; **329**: 821–30.
12. Oudega R, Hoes AW, Moons KGM. The Well's Rule does not adequately rule out deep vein thrombosis in primary care patients. *Ann Intern Med* 2005; **153**: 100–7.

13. Büller HR, Cate-Hoek AJT, Hoes AW, *et al.* Safely ruling out deep vein thrombosis in primary care. *Ann Intern Med* 2009; **150**: 229–35.

14. Kendall J, Reeves B, Clancy M. Point of care testing: randomised controlled trial of clinical outcome. *BMJ* 1998; **316**: 1052–7.

15. Crook M. *Handbook of near-patient testing.* Oxford: Oxford University Press, 1999.

16. Bjerrum L, Gahrn-Hansen B, Munck AP. C-reactive protein measurement in general practice may lead to lower antibiotic prescribing for sinusitis. *Brit J Gen Pract* 2004; **54**: 659–62.

17. Murphy MJ. Point of care testing: no pain, no gain. *Q J Med* 2001; **94**: 571–3.

18. Boucot KR, Seidman H, Weiss W. The Philadelphia pulmonary neoplasm research project. *Envir Res* 1977; **13**: 451–69.

19. Turkington PM, Kennan N, Greenstone MA. Misinterpretation of the chest X-ray as a factor in the delayed diagnosis of lung cancer. *Postgrad Med J* 2002; **78**: 158–60.

20. Balabanova Y, Coker R, Fedorin I, *et al.* Variability in interpretation of chest radiographs among Russian clinicians and implications for screening programmes: observational study. BMJ 2005; **331**: 379–82.

21. Buenger RE. Five thousand acute care/emergency department chest radiographs: comparison of requisitions with radiographic findings. *J Emerg Med* 1988; **6**: 197–202.

22. Logan JA, Vallance R, Willaims BO, *et al.* Does the chest x-ray alter the management of new patients attending a geriatric day hospital? *Health Bulletin* 1997; **55**: 52–7.

23. Pisarik P, Montoya C, Malloy ED. Clinical enquiries. When should a chest x-ray be used to evaluate acute-onset productive cough in adults? *JFam Pract* 2005; **54**: 1081–3.

24. Badgett RG, Mulrow CD, Otto PM, *et al.* How well can the chest radiograph diagnose left ventricular dysfunction? *J Gen Intern Med* 1996; **11**: 625–34.

25. Davenport C, Cheng EYL, Kwok YTT, *et al.* Assessing the diagnostic test accuracy of natriuretic peptides and ECG in the diagnosis of left ventricular systolic dysfunction: a systematic review and meta-analysis. *Brit J Gen Pract* 2006; **56**: 48–56.

26. Master SS, Longstreth GF, Liu AL. Results of computed tomography in family practitioners' patients with non-acute abdominal pain. *Family Practice* 2005; **22**: 474–7.

27. Jarvik JG, Deyo RA. Diagnostic evaluation of low back pain with emphasis on imaging. *Ann Intern Med* 2002; **137**: 586–97.

28. Summerton N, Paes R, Parker J. Patient specific deterrents and general practitioner referral for radiographic examination: a comparison between two distinct general practice communities. *J Clin Effect* 1998; **3**: 64–6.

29. Winkens RAG, Ament AJHA, Pop P, *et al.* Routine individual feedback on requests for diagnostic tests: an economic evaluation. *Med Decis Making* 1996; **16**: 309–14.

30. Winkens RAG, Grol RPTM, Beusmans GHMI, *et al.* Does a reduction in general practitioners' use of diagnostic tests lead to more hospital referrals? *Brit J Gen Pract* 1995; **45**: 289–92.

CHAPTER 8

Diagnostic research

INTRODUCTION

Primary care diagnostics should be based on the best available scientific evidence. This does not mean that such evidence is the only issue that matters: as emphasised in Chapter 2, clinical experience is also a critical component of the primary care diagnostic approach. However, in the absence of good quality research there is a risk that our diagnostic decision making is inefficient or inaccurate. We might also lose confidence in the value of the information obtained directly from the patient by means of the history or the examination. This chapter focuses on identification, appraisal, execution and application of primary care oriented diagnostic research.

FORMULATING THE QUESTION(S)

There are two broad types of question that need to be considered in seeking to research primary care diagnostics: clinical questions and processing questions.

Clinical questions

Formulating an answerable clinical question is critical to generating any data on the predictive validity of clinical information in addition to identifying work that has already been undertaken by other researchers. Such clinical questions comprise three core elements:

- the patient and their problem
- the intervention
- the patient-oriented outcome.

Occasionally there might be an additional requirement to consider a comparison intervention by, for example, contrasting the current diagnostic approach with a new strategy.

The patient-problem dyad is essentially synonymous with the iatrotropic complaint presenting to the primary care clinician. Examples include men over the age of 60 with bright red rectal bleeding, women between the ages of 20 and 40 years with dizziness, all individuals with new-onset palpitations or patients with iron-deficiency anaemia. Likewise the intervention equates with the clinical information subsequently extracted from the patient such as the further, more detailed description about the iatrotropic complaint, any associated symptoms and clinical features, the past medical history, the clinical examination and data obtained as a result of investigations.

Primary care diagnostics is also not simply about seeking to make a disease-oriented diagnosis, but about focusing on outcomes that matter to the patient. These might be not only mortality and morbidity but also discomfort, distress, dissatisfaction and a range of other patient-specific concerns. Reassuring a patient that they might not have cancer may be important but the detailed investigation of a benign rash for which no specific treatment is available can simply generate unnecessary distress and discomfort. Thus, from the patient's perspective, the clinical research question must be worth asking and the answer must be worth getting. Five particular issues about the outcomes should therefore be considered.

1 Is there an effective treatment for the target condition?
2 Could improved diagnosis result in either better treatment delivery or shorter treatment delay?
3 Would intervention at an earlier stage in the disease result in lowered mortality?
4 Would better diagnosis result in lowered morbidity both from the disease *and* from the diagnostic process?
5 How would improved diagnosis impact on patient-oriented outcomes?

Unfortunately a considerable volume of diagnostic research focuses on test-centred or disease-centred clinical questions. Although such evidence may furnish us with some helpful background information it is insufficient on its own.

Processing questions

In adopting a primary care approach it is important to have robust information in relation to the concurrent validity and the reliability of the clinical information being used. Furthermore, in order to adopt the Bayesian strategy we also require data about the prior probability (or prior odds) of the target disorder(s).

$$posterior\ odds = likelihood\ ratio \times prior\ odds$$

In common with predictive validity, reliability is population specific and needs to be studied in the setting where the clinical indicants will eventually be used. A common approach is to repeat the question after a time interval (intra-observer reliability) or for different examiners to assess the same patient (inter-observer reliability).

In generating information on concurrent validity or prior probability a comparison is generally made against a reference standard approximating to the 'truth'. Sackett *et al.* have produced some helpful guidance to appraise a report about prior probabilities (*see* Box 8.1).[1]

Box 8.1 Appraising a report about prior probabilities

1 Is this evidence about prior probabilities valid?
- Did the study patients represent the full spectrum of those who present with this clinical problem?
- Were the criteria for each final diagnosis explicit and credible?
- Was the diagnostic work-up comprehensive and consistently applied?
- For initially undiagnosed patients, was follow-up sufficiently long and complete?

2 Is this evidence about prior probabilities important?
- What were the diagnoses and their probabilities?
- How precise were these estimates of disease probability?

LITERATURE SEARCHING

Once a clinical question has been formulated, the next step is to identify the evidence to seek to answer the question. The search strategies shown in Table 8.1 exhibit reasonable accuracy in identifying published research (as assessed by their sensitivity and specificity) using Medline.[2]

EXECUTION OF DIAGNOSTIC RESEARCH

In generating indicants to support diagnosis in primary care settings two broad study designs have been adopted: case-control and cross-sectional. The case-control approach starts from the disease whereas the cross-sectional approach commences with the patient and their problem.

Case-control approach

Especially in recent years there has been a growing interest in the use of the case-control approach to generate clinical indicants.[3] In this study design subjects are

TABLE 8.1 Diagnostic search strategies in Medline

Search strategy	Sensitivity (%)	Specificity (%)
Sensitivity and specificity (exploded) *and* Specificity (text word)	71	99
Sensitivity and specificity (exploded) *and* Specificity (text word) *and* False-negative (text word)	73	98
Sensitivity and specificity (exploded) *and* Specificity (text word) *and* False-negative (text word) *and* Accuracy (text word)	80	97
Sensitivity and specificity (exploded) *and* Specificity (text word) *and* False-negative (text word) *and* Accuracy (text word) *and* Screening (text word)	89	92

selected on the basis of whether they do (cases) or do not (controls) have a particular disease under study. Data are then extracted (retrospectively) in order to seek to assess the diagnostic value of clinical information. The major advantage of such a study design is that it is relatively quick and inexpensive compared with the cross-sectional approach (especially if the latter also incorporates a period of prospective patient follow-up in order to establish the reference diagnosis) and is said to be particularly helpful in the study of the diagnosis of rare diseases such as cancer.[4]

As discussed earlier my colleagues and I have used the case-control design in order to seek to assess the potential clinical value of the patient's pattern of attendance in relation to cancer diagnosis.[5] The method initially involved identifying 83 patients with cancer by means of an extensive search of the patient information systems in my own practice, supplemented by an internal practice notification system. Using the practice's computerised patient database, each of these cancer cases was then matched (using age, gender and postcode) to two non-cancer controls. This process gave rise to 249 observations (i.e. 83 matched sets).

Using a standard proforma, two examinations were then made of all written records by a researcher and a medical practitioner in order to identify any consultations (at the main/branch surgery or as a result of a home visit) with the GP for the three years preceding the date of diagnosis (or pseudo-diagnosis). The date of diagnosis was defined as the earliest date of 'specialist' confirmation (ideally by histology *but* alternatively by radiology, cytology or biochemistry). For the controls a pseudo-diagnostic date was defined as the date at which the control's age exactly equalled that for the appropriate case.

For all controls and cases information was specifically sought on the following potential confounders with a view to adjusting for them in the analysis: smoking status, occupation and marital status. In order to address the issue of co-morbidity increasing the consultation rate, the *dominant function* of each consultation was also dichotomised into new problem or follow-up/preventative/administrative/other. Acute exacerbations of a chronic disease such as a severe worsening of asthma requiring oral steroids were also defined as new problems.

More recently Hamilton *et al.* have undertaken a series of much larger case-control studies looking at the symptomatic diagnosis of cancer in primary care.[6,7] In their study of colorectal cancer, for example, their cases and controls were drawn from 21 practices in Exeter, UK. The total recruitment amounted to 349 patients with colorectal cancer (identified by means of the local cancer registry) and 1744 controls matched by age, sex and general practice. Furthermore, the full medical record for 2 years before diagnosis was coded using the International Classification of Primary Care-2.

However, for the primary care clinician the most obvious problem with the case-control approach is that it is disease-oriented rather than patient-oriented. Thus, although Hamilton *et al.* have produced a very helpful list of symptoms associated with colorectal cancer and their predictive values, they could not distinguish between the iatrotropic and the non-iatrotropic information. Without an understanding about what actually brought the patient to the doctor in the first instance (i.e. the prior probability) it is difficult for the primary care clinician to rationally incorporate such information into their daily practice.

A related issue is that the case-control approach is exclusive rather than inclusive. In a recent review of a large number of diagnostic studies it was concluded that, generally, case-control studies overestimated predictive validity.[8] Compared with cross-sectional studies that recruited a group of patients unselected by disease status and representative of the population in which the clinical indicant(s) was to be used, the relative diagnostic odds was inflated three-fold within the case-control studies. This may be due to case-control researchers omitting cases from their study groups that were mild, uncertain or difficult to diagnose.

There are some more detailed methodological concerns that can, in some circumstances, cast doubt on the applicability of the case-control approach to patient-centred diagnostic research.

The study population

Traditionally many case-control studies were undertaken amongst groups of hospital patients. However, as a general practitioner I know that I am considerably more likely to admit patients with certain combinations of clinical information and this may distort the clinical indicant values derived from studies in such hospital populations.[9] For example, respiratory and orthopaedic conditions are not associated in the general population but a strong link has been demonstrated in hospital. Similarly laxative use and arthritic disease have been observed to have a strong relationship in hospital patients, which is quite different from that found outside hospitals.

Another major concern about the case-control approach is that it generally relies on prevalent (existing) rather than incident (new-onset) cases. Working backwards to obtain data on potential clinical indicants may be difficult due to the time lapse with individuals having moved or died. For example, although the incidence rate of colorectal cancer is slightly higher in males than in females, the survival from colorectal cancer is longer in women than in men. Thus in a case-control study using prevalent cases of colorectal cancer there will be a higher proportion of women than in a corresponding sample of incident cases.

The clinical information

My experience of undertaking case-control studies has taught me that one of the greatest difficulties encountered is the inaccessibility or inadequacy of routine medical records. Records may be lost, information may be accidentally (or deliberately!) mis-recorded, and key clinical information might be recorded in different places and in a variety of formats. In our case-control study we did not consider telephone contacts or consultations and contacts with practice nurses and other professional/administrative staff. Attendances at other NHS portals outside the practice, e.g.

secondary care or 'emergency/temporary' visits to other general practices (e.g. during holidays) were also excluded.[5]

Even as a primary care clinician interested in diagnostic research I know that on a day-to-day basis I struggle to record sufficient data (and in a consistent format) that would satisfy me as a clinical researcher. I also have no idea about what information a future case-control researcher struggling to read through my clinical records in 10 years time might find helpful or what precise question they may be attempting to answer. In seeking to use routine primary care clinical records to undertake diagnostic research, it seems that some rather over-optimistic assumptions are being made about the quality of the data recorded. In our case-control study we specifically focused on the pattern of attendance as we considered that these sorts of data were likely to exhibit considerably more robustness than information on other aspects of the past medical history. However, when we sought to consider the potential confounders, there were certainly problems with missing data: no information was available on smoking status for five patients and occupation for 22 patients.[5]

It is also particularly easy to be misled by written records concerning particular symptoms. As discussed in Chapter 4 there is considerable inter- and intra-doctor and patient variability in symptom definitions. Furthermore, in relation to colorectal cancer diagnosis, an early symptom such as a slight change in bowel habit, some mild abdominal pain or a feeling of general malaise might lead to the patient purchasing an over-the-counter remedy or changing their diet. Such adjustments can modify the presentation of the original symptom(s) or even produce new symptoms. Several years later it will be impossible to ascertain which of the symptoms identified from the retrospective scrutiny of records are 'primary symptoms' and which are consequent upon some other intervening factor.

From the primary care perspective the case-control design also does not permit the assessment of the predictive validity of new or 'non-traditional' clinical information. Although we might *now* be interested in certain clinical information to help us to achieve a diagnosis, this may not have been the case several years ago. Consequently the recording of such information would have been accorded a low priority by a busy clinician and a case-control study examining their records several years later might conclude (erroneously) that the clinical information is of little value. At a broader level it is worth re-emphasising that primary care diagnostics is about acknowledging that the reporting and the recording of symptoms cannot be considered in isolation from either the patient's co-existing medical and social circumstances or the doctor's consultation style.

In adopting a primary care approach to diagnosis I would argue that clinical indicants derived from case-control studies should be handled with great care. Personally I believe that the primary role of the case-control approach should be to provide information to guide the future development of well-conducted cross-sectional studies. For example, in relation to the earlier diagnosis of colorectal cancer, a case-control approach could provide some valuable insights into clinical indicant differences between late and early stage cancers. Nesting a case-control study within a prospective cohort might also overcome some concerns about the representative nature of the study population.

Cross-sectional approach

A cross-sectional study seeks to compare items (or combinations of items) of clinical information against a 'reference standard' within a pre-defined group of patients.[10] Where follow-up is used this is to develop or enhance the validity of the reference standard (e.g. 'delayed-type' cross-sectional studies where the reference standard diagnosis is arrived at after a pre-determined period of follow-up). Above all the study group should be defined by the iatrotropic symptom or abnormality that would cause a patient to consult their primary care clinician.

In designing robust cross-sectional studies a number of key issues need to be considered.

Defining the study population

Our new-onset palpitation study sought to explore the generation of clinical indicants in the setting where they would be used by general practitioners.[11] A network of 62 general practitioners spread amongst 36 practices agreed to recruit patients with new-onset palpitations over the course of a 9-month study period. Patients consenting to be involved in the study were asked a number of questions, focusing particularly on patient characteristics and the medical history and were also requested to complete a 'Hospital Anxiety and Depression Scale'. Each patient was provided with a 'RhythmCard' cardiac event recorder for up to 2 weeks (the reference standard) and was asked to record their heart rhythm if they experienced palpitations.

Unfortunately, selection bias is often a major problem in studies that rely on the recruitment of patients by primary care clinicians. A general practitioner with an average list size of 2000 patients would expect to see six patients with palpitations per year.[12] Consequently, the 62 general practitioners involved in the study over a 9-month period should have recruited 279 patients and yet only 139 were entered into the study.

Primary care clinicians may only recruit patients into research studies that they would have referred onwards anyway, e.g. patients with moderate symptoms of prostatism might only be included in a study of such symptoms if they have also been noted to have an enlarged prostate (selection by test outcome). In different situations there may be a tendency to enlist patients with intermediate or greater probabilities of illness (selection by clinical spectrum). Patients with significant co-morbidities might also be excluded from many such diagnostic studies and the range of differential diagnoses in the study population may consequently not reflect the true situation in primary care.

One possible way to address such selection bias is to undertake more careful scrutiny of the primary care clinicians. This approach has been used with some limited success by Fijten *et al.* in a small subset of practices in the context of a larger study of patients presenting with rectal bleeding.[13] However, it was seen as extremely difficult and costly to develop this process on a broader scale.

In our new-onset haematuria study we explored a different approach by using an open-access clinic as a proxy setting for macroscopic haematuria presenting to the general practitioner.[14] However, it remains a matter of judgement as to how representative the study population is likely to be in relation to all the haematuria patients encountered within primary care. Particular concerns are referral bias by general practitioners selectively sending patients into the clinic and, even once a referral is made, some patients may die or move away from the area during the time in which they are waiting to attend the clinic. Furthermore, not all patients entering secondary care with haematuria will be caught by an open-access system; there are other ports of entry from primary care for haematuria patients such as via the renal physicians or as an emergency with, perhaps, renal colic.

In a study of the diagnosis of carpal tunnel syndrome we undertook a community survey to bypass the general practitioner in order to artificially construct a 'clinically relevant' population (defined as those with 'unpleasant tingling sensations, numbness or both in their fingers or hands' who have consulted or felt that they should consult their doctor). Our closely related study of symptoms of possible oncological significance used the same approach and also provides some further reassurance that such a community-based mechanism can produce reliable symptom-defined groupings that are not dramatically dissimilar from those identified by others.[15] We have also established that the apparently simple question 'have you consulted or would you consider consulting your doctor about ...?' seems to be a reasonable assessment of an individual's consulting behaviour in relation to a specific symptom.

In developing this work further we plan to examine the potential of using waiting-room surveys to complement the community-based or physician-notification approaches. Attending the waiting room may indicate something about the general healthcare seeking behaviour of patients and, furthermore, waiting room surveys also represent an opportunity to check for selection bias in relation to doctor notification of symptoms.

In generating clinical indicants applicable to primary care decision making it may be that the main approach (dictated by the defining symptom) requires supporting by a second arm in a different setting in order to address any particular methodological concerns. For example, although an open-access endoscopy clinic may be a particularly appropriate primary care proxy for patients over the age of 50 with new-onset dyspepsia, some additional work will need to be undertaken amongst patients presenting directly to a small group of primary care clinicians. This is to ensure that the doctors are referring an appropriate patient spectrum in the 'correct' fashion and not selecting particular groups of individuals for referral directly to a gastroenterologist or a surgeon, bypassing the open-access clinic completely.

One remaining concern about using a symptom to define a study group relates to symptom characterisation. There is a need to ensure that the key defining question (i.e. 'do you have unpleasant tingling sensations, numbness or both in your fingers or hands?' in the context of our carpal tunnel syndrome study) is the most appropriate in order to identify an epidemiologically useful grouping to refine diagnostic discrimination in primary care settings. As symptoms are rarely synonymous with a single condition, careful consideration needs to be given to striking a sensible balance between the defining symptom specificity (with the possibility of over-inclusion) and sensitivity (with the potential for under-inclusion).

In primary care settings a further difficulty is that, although some patients may present with symptoms that are clear-cut such as an irregular heart rate, others may consult their doctor with vague complaints such as a 'fluttering' sensation in the epigastrium. In the latter case the primary care physician seeking to use the clinical indicants from a new-onset palpitation study will need to judge how closely the patients in the study population match up to the patient who is sitting in their consulting room. Future work will also need to move beyond the easily characterised symptoms (e.g. macroscopic haematuria) in order to define study groupings in relation to some of the vague presentations, such as tiredness or general malaise.

Clearly some problems will never easily fit into any inception grouping and in these circumstances doctors working in primary care become more dependent on information elicited from direct patient questioning. The community-based surveillance approach has the added bonus of providing information on the discriminant value of, for example, rectal bleeding, abdominal pain or change in normal bowel habit in patients who choose to consult their general practitioner about the symptom (i.e. an iatrotropic symptom), *in addition* to information on the discriminant value of symptoms that patients experience but do not lead them to consult (non-iatrotropic symptoms). This latter information may be particularly applicable to direct patient questioning when there is no clearly identifiable iatrotropic symptom.

Generating the clinical indicants

When a patient attends their primary care physician with an iatrotropic symptom, the general practitioner might simply act on the basis of the information that has been presented (e.g. by initiating a referral or offering reassurance). However, it is more likely that the doctor will attempt to obtain further details in order to reach a better understanding of the patient's presentation. As discussed earlier this process might involve clarification of the nature of the presenting symptom and/or seeking additional clinical data as well as information about the individual and their past history. Thus, in keeping with the primary care physician's clinical approach, once a symptom-related study population has been defined, the next research step is to decide what further information needs to be obtained and how this process should be undertaken.

In our new-onset palpitation, new-onset haematuria and community-based studies we focused exclusively on patient characteristics and the medical history.[11,14,15] The question selection was determined by a combination of accepted clinical practice and, where possible, the adoption of previously used instruments. However, there may be other features of a patient's presentation that have discriminant value and, in some circumstances, case-control studies could be used to explore the potential value of a more novel piece of clinical information, such as the patient's pattern of surgery attendance.[5]

Qualitative research amongst patients, relatives and general practitioners offers another possible avenue to identify potential clinical indicants worthy of further study. Salander *et al.* used interviews of a consecutive sample of 28 patients with malignant gliomas and their spouses in order to enquire about symptom development and help-seeking behaviour.[16] Their detailed work highlighted the high prevalence of mental symptoms, such as fatigue and irritation in the time prior to definitive diagnosis.

Measuring change is an important additional type of information that primary care clinicians often rely on in their decision making. The intention is to distinguish between those individuals who change a lot and those who change little. Unfortunately directly asking questions about change (i.e. assessing responsiveness) in a cross-sectional study is fraught with errors and the preferred approach is to directly measure the attribute at the beginning of the study period and at appropriate intervals thereafter.

Once there is clarity about the information that will be sought there is a further requirement to be confident about the means by which the information is actually elicited. In our new-onset palpitation study the additional data were extracted by general practitioners with the aid of a questionnaire, in our new-onset haematuria study nurse practitioners obtained the information using a modified audit proforma, and in our carpal tunnel study the process was undertaken by a non-primary care doctor using a primary care-oriented questionnaire. Finally, in the community-based study of symptoms of possible oncological significance the task was shared between three primary care-oriented Medical Research Council-trained research nurses under the guidance of a general practitioner and using a primary care-oriented data collection instrument.

As discussed in Chapter 4, the extraction of clinical information from a patient involves a complex interaction with their physician and seeking to mimic this process in the context of a research study is extremely difficult. Although using general practitioners would be the ideal, our choice of the nurse-oriented approach for the community-based cancer symptom study was dictated by concerns of cost and data completeness. However, although I have reasonable confidence in their substitution for general practitioners in the context of this study, it is clear that if primary care-trained and oriented research nurses are going to be used in future studies as proxies for general practitioners then a more formal comparison with primary care physicians will need to be undertaken.

Selecting the reference standard

In all cross-sectional diagnostic analytical studies, the method to identify clinical indicants involves undertaking a comparison of the clinical information against the 'truth' (the reference standard).[10] In our new-onset palpitation, new-onset haematuria and carpal tunnel studies we sought to use reference standards (i.e. 'RhythmCard', cystoscopy/ultrasound, and electrophysiology respectively) that approximated the 'truth' as far as possible in keeping with the realities of primary care clinical decision making. Thus for conditions that might lead to referral (i.e. urological malignancies and significant arrhythmias) we selected reference standards that would lead to less precise action-related dichotomous diagnoses. For carpal tunnel syndrome we were more concerned with precision as, unlike urological malignancy, this is a condition that can sometimes be managed adequately in primary care. However, in developing the community-based approach to cancer diagnosis further within a large number of practices, considerations of cost as well as the invasive and potentially hazardous nature of any investigations (e.g. colonoscopy) will become key considerations in selecting an appropriate reference standard. In these circumstances an alternative approach could involve determining the 'truth' by careful observation over a pre-defined period.

During 1989, 933 patients with new-onset non-acute abdominal complaints within Limburg, Holland were recruited by local general practitioners.[17] All patients underwent a physical examination by their general practitioner, were asked to complete a questionnaire on symptoms/psychological factors and were subjected to some simple investigations. The patients' records were subsequently reviewed after 1 year in order to assess the nature of the final diagnosis. Information was then provided on which symptoms and signs were most helpful in predicting which of the patients with non-acute abdominal symptoms at one point subsequently turned out to have serious disease.

An ideal study of diagnosis in primary care using 'pathology at follow-up' as the reference standard, would adopt a study design that closely reflected the natural history of patient follow-up in primary care. Three to four weekly reassessments (if possible combined with symptom diaries) of patients would not only provide some very useful information on the measurement of change but it would also enable the study to assess in a more rigorous fashion the association between the clinical information and the eventual diagnosis. In the absence of a clear link between the symptoms and the outcome, the extent of misclassification bias is very dependent on the length of follow-up. If the observation period is too short conditions may be missed; too long and false linkages may be construed between symptoms and outcomes. Detection bias is a related problem resulting from, for example, preferential referral of patients with abdominal pain and rectal bleeding as opposed to abdominal pain alone. Thus an early cancer may be more likely to be detected in a patient with abdominal pain and rectal bleeding than in a patient solely with abdominal pain. Clearly, the length of follow-up also needs to be designed to address this issue.

Finally, there may be pathological and clinical indicant dissimilarities in the presentation of patients who develop definitive disease after a shorter period of observation and there may be a requirement for time-specific stratification of the reference standard categorisation.

Either through losses to follow-up in delayed-type cross-sectional studies, or resource constraints in the case of other reference standards, only a proportion of individuals may be subjected to the gold standard. To avoid so-called verification or work-up bias it is essential that every individual (or a representative random selection of sufficient power) from whom clinical information is extracted are also submitted for assessment by the reference standard. If this does not occur there tends to be an overestimate of the strength of the association.[18]

It is well recognised that knowledge of clinical or other factors can, in certain circumstances, influence a diagnostic test result. Thus if the reference standard involves an interpretable component, it is important that it is assessed independently and, if possible, blind in relation to the clinical information already obtained. In our carpal tunnel and new-onset palpitation studies the reference standards were assessed independently, in the new-onset haematuria study the clinic-based reference standard (using cystoscopy and ultrasonography) was supplemented by an independent examination of the patient records 2–3 months later.

In all diagnostic research, the underlying assumption is that there really is an identifiable truth; a diagnostic category that fits the clinical information and that such a diagnosis can be verified by an independent reference standard method. Unfortunately, this may not be the case and, in the absence of an adequate reference standard, statistical methods are being developed in order to estimate the accuracy of new tests. There may even need to be a re-assessment of the nature of diagnostic reference standards in primary care oriented diagnostic research with, perhaps, more of an emphasis on the diagnosis of 'wellness' by using a battery of reference standards to exclude serious or important illness (reverse reference standard) or even reference standards related to a course of action rather than a clinical diagnosis. For example, McWhinney has suggested that the division of headaches into sumatriptan responsive and non-sumatriptan responsive might be more appropriate in primary care than the traditional dichotomy between tension headaches and migraines.[19]

Establishing a link

In deciding on the significance of a possible link between the clinical information and a reference standard, it is not necessary to demonstrate causality but rather a strong association. However, in primary care where there is a greater reliance on surrogate makers of potential disease it is important to be clear about what information has been considered within a study and what has not.

The importance of statistical significance is overplayed in many diagnostic studies. According to Deeks, for a diagnostic marker to be clinically useful, the relationship between the marker and the disease has to be very strong. Therefore, unless sample sizes are very small, it is unlikely that clinically important results are also not statistically significant.[20]

APPLICATION OF PRIMARY CARE-ORIENTED DIAGNOSTIC RESEARCH

Whatever educational, guideline or decision-support initiatives are developed for primary care clinicians (and those training to be primary care clinicians) these must be built on high quality evidence that more explicitly considers the primary care perspective. A further requirement is to focus downstream from the clinical indicant in order to assess its influence on subsequent patient management, patient-oriented outcomes and the eventual course of the clinical condition.

Engaging the primary care clinician

Once an indicant has been generated it needs to be made available to the primary care clinician in a useable format. Even the best clinical indicants may fail to have any impact as they may be inaccessible in form or place of publication. Ways need to be found to ensure that the information in peer-reviewed journals is available to all primary care clinicians. If the clinical indicants are published in relatively obscure places, primary care physicians will simply not have the time or inclination to search them out. Furthermore, if doctors also believe that there is no relevant information available that could assist them with their diagnostic decision making they will not even make the effort to look for it.

A Bayesian-type approach to applying clinical indicants is favoured in this book.

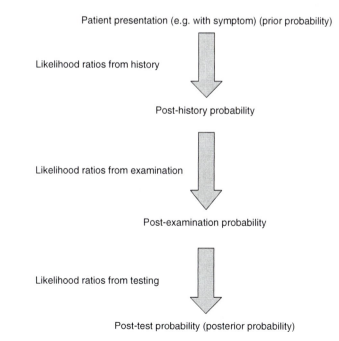

Although this seems to accord with the hypothetico-deductive approach to clinical decision making, general practitioners may make errors in the estimation of the pre-test probability (also referred to as inappropriate setting of the anchor; *see* Chapter 2) by failing to properly consider the prevalence of the target disorder in the population they are assessing. Furthermore, in a recent survey amongst Swiss general practitioners, although many respondents recognised the correct definitions for the common discriminant terms they were often applied incorrectly.[21]

Elstein and Schwarz[22] argue that clinicians trained in methods of evidence-based medicine are more likely than untrained clinicians to use a Bayesian approach to interpret findings. Thus if newer indicants are going to refine diagnostic discrimination in primary care settings then any research findings must also be linked to education in relation to clinical decision making.

Incorporating clinical indicants into clinical practice

In evaluating the application of clinical indicants into general practice we might be interested in a number of issues.

1. Is this diagnostic approach 'better' than the existing diagnostic approach?
2. Is this diagnostic sequence or package 'better' than an alternative sequence or package?
3. Is this overall diagnostic strategy 'better' than the current approach?
4. What is the added value of further and/or more invasive testing?

However, from the patient's perspective 'better' might be more about effectiveness, equity, appropriateness, acceptability and accessibility rather than cost-effectiveness or efficiency. Moreover, there is a requirement to distinguish the short-term from the long-term outcomes and to consider what level of uncertainty and imprecision can be accommodated by the patient (and the doctor).

In assessing the applicability of clinical indicants one sequence is illustrated by the development of the 'Ottawa ankle rules' for acute ankle injuries. In 1992 Stiell *et al.* undertook a study of 750 emergency department patients over a 5-month period. They surveyed for 32 standardised clinical variables that were compared against a radiographic gold standard in order to develop clinical indicants for malleolar fractures. Such fractures were more likely to be identified among people who had pain near the malleoli and who were aged 55 years or more, had localised bone tenderness of the posterior edge or tip of either malleolus, or were unable to bear weight both immediately after the injury and in the emergency department.[23]

These indicants were subsequently prospectively evaluated and refined in a second study amongst a new set of patients.[24] A final study sought to use a controlled trial in order to assess the feasibility and impact of introducing the indicants (combined together as a clinical decision rule – the 'Ottawa ankle rules') to a large number of physicians in the emergency departments of eight teaching and community hospitals in Canada.[25] This work demonstrated that the use of the 'Ottawa ankle rules' led to reductions in the use of ankle radiography, waiting times and costs without an increased number of missed malleolar fractures.

When the 'Ottawa ankle rules' were published they were set with a sensitivity of 100% as it was thought that many clinicians would be reluctant to use the rules if there were any false-negative results. Similarly, in generating clinical indicants (or clinical decision rules) in order to refine diagnostic discrimination in primary care there is a need to establish the level of false-positive and false-negative diagnoses that primary care clinicians and their patients are willing to accept.

According to Laupacis et al.[26] the likelihood that clinical indicants and clinical decision rules will be used by doctors is increased if they make clinical sense, are easy to use and suggest a course of action rather than simply a disease probability. The success of the 'Ottawa ankle rules' has been attributed to the rigour within which they were derived and tested combined with their clinical sensibility in that no obvious items were missing and that the method of aggregating component variables was reasonable. Consideration was also given to the time to apply the rule and the ease of use, factors of equal relevance to the generation of clinical indicants for use by primary care clinicians (*see also* Chapter 3).

The ankle rule sequence of developing, validating and implementing points the way for much future research in relation to primary care diagnostics. However, in view of the costs of such studies I believe it is also necessary to develop a prioritisation framework evaluating any new diagnostic tool as shown in Box 8.2.

Box 8.2 Suggested prioritisation criteria for evaluating any new diagnostic tool for possible use with primary care[27,28]

The disease or target condition	– Can the disease or target condition to which the new tool will be applied be clearly defined?
	– Is the disease or target condition an important problem in terms of prevalence/incidence or morbidity/mortality?
	– Is the disease or target condition a regional or national priority?
	– Does the disease or target condition present a diagnostic problem (i.e. inaccuracy or inefficiency) and would it be useful to have better diagnostic tools?
	– Is there variation in treatment or patient outcomes resulting from current diagnostic variability?
	– Could the diagnostic processing pathway for the disease or target condition be improved by obtaining information in a less risky fashion or in a manner more acceptable to patients?

The new diagnostic tool being considered (such as developments in the history and examination, clinical decision/prediction rules, pathology, genetics, physiological testing, imaging or endoscopy).	– Would the tool have a clearly defined role in the diagnostic pathway, e.g. replacing an existing test, as a triage tool, or after the diagnostic pathway as an add-on test? – Is it safe and acceptable to patients? – Does the new tool have the potential to improve the ability to confirm or rule out the disease or target condition? – Would the new tool enhance diagnostic efficiency and/or be more cost-effective than the current approach? – Would it be feasible to assess the validity and the reliability of the new technology within primary care? – Would it be straightforward to change current practice to incorporate this tool (for example by introducing additional requirements for training, infrastructure and quality control)?
The impact of better diagnosis	– Is there an effective treatment for the disease or target condition and could improved diagnosis lead to either better treatment delivery or reduced treatment delay? Is there the potential for decreases in workload and costs? – Would intervention at an earlier stage in the disease or target condition result in lowered mortality? – Would better diagnosis result in lowered morbidity both from the disease or target condition and from the diagnostic process?

GENERAL REFERENCES

- Armstrong BK, White E, Saracci R. *Principles of Exposure Measurement in Epidemiology*. Oxford: Oxford University Press, 1992.
- Fletcher RH, Fletcher SW, Wagner EH. *Clinical Epidemiology: the essentials*. Baltimore: Williams & Wilkins, 1996.
- Sackett DL, Haynes RB, Guyatt GH, *et al*. *Clinical Epidemiology: a basic science for clinical medicine*. Boston: Little, Brown and Company, 1991.
- Streiner DL, Norman GR. *Health Measurement Scales*. Oxford: Oxford University Press, 1995.

TEXT REFERENCES

1. Sackett DL, Strauss SE, Richardson WS. *Evidence-Based Medicine: how to practise and teach EBM*. London: Churchill Livingstone, 2000.
2. Deville WLJM, Bezemer PD, Bouter LM. Publications on diagnostic test evaluation in family medicine journals: an optimal search strategy. *J Clin Epidemiol* 2000; **53**: 65–9.
3. Herman JM. Case-control studies. *Fam Med* 1990; **22**: 52–5.
4. Friedman GD, Skilling JS, Udaltsova NV, *et al*. Early symptoms of ovarian cancer: a case-control study without recall bias. *Family Practice* 2005; **22**: 548–53.
5. Summerton N, Rigby AS, Mann S, *et al*. The general practitioner–patient consultation pattern as a tool for cancer diagnosis in general practice. *Brit J Gen Pract* 2003; **53**: 50–2.
6. Hamilton W, Peters TJ, Round A, *et al*. What are the clinical features of lung cancer before the diagnosis is made? A population based case-control study. *Thorax* 2005; **60**: 1059–65.
7. Hamilton W, Round A, Sharp D, *et al*. Clinical features of colorectal cancer before diagnosis: a population-based case-control study. *Brit J Cancer* 2005; **93**: 399–405.
8. Lijmer JG, Mol BW, Heisterkamp S, *et al*. Empirical evidence of design-related bias in studies of diagnostic tests. *JAMA* 1999; **282**: 1061–6.
9. Sackett DL. Bias in analytic research. *J Chron Dis* 1979; **32**: 51–63.
10. Knottnerus JA, Muris JW. Assessment of the accuracy of diagnostic tests: the cross-sectional study. *J Clin Epidemiol* 2003; **56**: 1118–28.
11. Summerton N, Mann S, Rigby AS, *et al*. New onset palpitations in general practice: assessing the discriminant value of items within the clinical history. *Family Practice* 2001; **18**: 383–92.
12. Zwietering PJ, Knottnerus JA, Rinkens PELM, *et al*. Arrhythmias in general practice: diagnostic value of patient characteristics, medical history and symptoms. *Family Practice* 1998; **15**: 343–53.
13. Fijten GH, Starmans R, Muris JWM, *et al*. Predictive value of signs and symptoms for colorectal cancer in patients with rectal bleeding in general practice. *Family Practice* 1995; **12**: 279–86.
14. Summerton N, Mann S, Rigby AS, *et al*. Patients with new onset haematuria: assessing the discriminant value of items of clinical information in relation to urological malignancies. *Brit J Gen Pract* 2002; **52**: 284–9.
15. Summerton N, Mann S, Sutton J, *et al*. Developing clinically relevant and reproducible symptom-defined populations for cancer diagnostic research in general practice using a community survey. *Family Practice* 2003; **20**: 340–6.
16. Salander P, Bergenheim AT, Hamberg K, *et al*. Pathways from symptoms to medical care: a descriptive study of symptom development and obstacles to early diagnosis in brain tumour patients. *Family Practice* 1999; **16**: 143–8.
17. Muris J WM, Starmans R, Fijten GH, *et al*. Non-acute abdominal complaints in general practice: diagnostic value of signs and symptoms. *Brit J Gen Pract* 1995; **45**: 313–16.
18. Begg CB. Biases in the assessment of diagnostic tests. *Statistics in Medicine* 1987; **6**: 411–23.
19. McWhinney IR. *A Textbook of Family Medicine*. Oxford: Oxford University Press, 1997.

20. Deeks JJ. Using evaluations of diagnostic tests: understanding their limitations and making the most of available evidence. *Ann Oncol* 1999; **10**: 761–8.

21. Steurer J, Fischer JE, Bachmann LM, *et al.* Communicating accuracy of tests to general practitioners: a controlled study. *BMJ* 2002; **324**: 824–6.

22. Elstein AS, Schwarz A. Clinical problem solving and diagnostic decision making: selective review of the cognitive literature. *BMJ* 2002; **324**: 729–32.

23. Stiell IG, Greenberg GH, McKnight RD, *et al.* A study to develop clinical decision rules for the use of radiography in acute ankle injuries. *Annals of Emergency Medicine* 1992; **21**: 384–90.

24. Stiell IG, Greenberg GH, McKnight RD, *et al.* Decision rules for the use of radiography in acute ankle injuries. Refinement and prospective validation. *JAMA* 1993; **269**: 1127–32.

25. Stiell I, Wells G, Laupacis A, *et al.* Multicentre trial to introduce the Ottawa ankle rules for use of radiography in acute ankle injuries. *BMJ* 1995; **311**: 594–7.

26. Laupacis A, Sekar N, Stiell IG. Clinical prediction rules. A review and suggested modifications of methological standards. *JAMA* 1997; **277**: 488–94.

27. Summerton N. Selecting diagnostic tests for evaluation. *BMJ* 2008; **336**: 683.

28. Pluddermann A, Heneghan C, Thompson M, *et al.* Prioritisation criteria for the selection of new diagnostic technologies for evaluation (in press). *BMC Health Services Research* 2010; **10**: 109–119.

CHAPTER 9

The application of primary care diagnostics 1: cancer

Recognising cancer can be difficult. It is especially tricky in primary care where cancers are rare, there is a greater reliance on symptoms, and general practitioners are constantly bombarded with guidelines and initiatives that ignore the primary care context.

Nowadays I feel that I am forced to walk an increasingly thin tightrope, balancing the often-conflicting demands and expectations of patients, consultants, health authorities and professional organisations. Like most general practitioners I am always anxious to not miss a serious or important condition in a patient; on the other hand, I am aware of the need to avoid over-investigation or over-referral of patients. Both extremes are costly to the health service as a whole and can have significant adverse consequences for individual patients and their families.

It is now known that one out of every twenty encounters with a GP will involve patients exhibiting one of the seven warning signs of cancer.[1] Moreover, in general, the earlier that a cancer is diagnosed, the better is the prognosis.

Earlier recognition of colorectal cancer by general practitioners is often cited as a particular problem:

- Despite the reduction in the mortality rate over the last ten years, the long-term results of surgery in the UK remain disappointing. This is mainly due to the late/ advanced presentation of over one-quarter of colorectal cancers. There is some evidence that a reduction in the time between the onset of symptoms and referral to hospital by GPs results in an improvement in the Dukes' staging.[2]
- Comparison of colorectal cancer survival rates across Europe shows significant inter-country differences. It has been suggested that the poorer survival rates in the UK compared to those in some other parts of Western Europe are due to late presentation.[3]

	Eindhoven area	Thames area
Three year survival	55%	38%
Proportion of Dukes' A/B	55%	42%

Three-year survival and earlier Dukes' stages in two registry areas of Europe[3]

- 20–30% of patients with colorectal cancers present as emergencies with intestinal obstruction or, occasionally, perforation or bleeding. As such, patients are invariably frailer than they would have been had they presented earlier; the mortality in this group is considerably increased (postoperative mortality 19% compared to 8% in comparable elective cases). It has been suggested that such cases represent a marker for failure of adequate diagnostic assessment within primary care.[4] In a recent audit it was found that 63% of patients presenting as emergencies had reported at least one symptom to their doctors in the month before diagnosis.[5] Moreover, three symptoms seem to be particularly associated with an emergency presentation: abdominal pain (odds ratio 6.2), loss of weight (odds ratio 3.4) and diarrhoea (odds ratio 3.4).

My view is that general practitioners have an important role in earlier cancer recognition and, back in 1999, I wrote *'Diagnosing Cancer in Primary Care'* as a concise, primary care-based aid to clinical assessment by outlining epidemiological data, risk factors, symptoms and signs of the more common cancers, along with the place and value of investigations. However, a dozen years later, matters have become much more formalised and, as a general practitioner, I am now subject to a range of guidelines designed by non-clinical academics and cancer specialists. Consequently I think the time is ripe to re-assess the approach to cancer recognition within primary care in accordance with some of the principles outlined in this book.

MAINTAINING A BROAD PERSPECTIVE

Compared to 20 years ago, I seem to see a significant number of patients worried that their headache, wrist lump or dizziness has a more sinister aetiology than a migraine, ganglion or benign positional vertigo respectively. The primary care approach emphasises the need to think more broadly and to be aware that a patient presenting with a symptom of 'possible oncological significance' might have other conditions (both serious and not-so-serious) aside from cancer.

In Chapter 2 I discussed the idea that diagnostic decision making is often partially dependent on a number of heuristics, or 'rules of thumb', in order to recall or to understand knowledge – something that is especially relevant to the assessment of possible cancer symptoms. A failure to appreciate that we may be using such heuristics can result in important cognitive errors being made by clinicians working in a primary care context (where new cancers are rarely encountered) who have spent a significant period employed or studying in secondary or tertiary care settings (where whole clinics are full of patients with cancer). For example, GPs can easily produce a distorted range of differential diagnoses through failure to take into account the relative prevalence of conditions in a primary care setting, misassign probability estimates or judge the odds of an event by the ease with which it can be remembered.

TABLE 9.1 Diagnoses at three years after presentation with haematuria in general practice

Diagnosis at three years	Women (% of diagnoses)	Men (% of diagnoses)
Urinary tract cancer	3.7	8.0
Renal calculi	1.5	3.8
Urinary tract infection	34.7	20.6
Benign prostatic hypertrophy		7.3
Orchitis		2.6
Menstrual disorders	8.5	
Glomerulonephritis	0.1	0.2
Urethritis	0.1	0.4
Bleeding disorders	0.3	0.5
Polycystic kidneys	0.1	0.1
Infective endocarditis	0.1	0.0
Prostate cancer		3.1
Uterine cancer	0.4	

A recent study examining the diagnoses after 3 years of 762 325 individuals aged 15 years or older presenting to general practice with the objective symptoms of haematuria, haemoptysis or rectal bleeding provided the data in tables 9.1–9.3.[6]

The percentages in Tables 9.1–9.3 also represent positive predictive values (i.e. the probability that the disease is present if the patient has a particular symptom).

TABLE 9.2 Diagnoses at three years after presentation with haemoptysis in general practice

Diagnosis at three years	Women (% of diagnoses)	Men (% of diagnoses)
Lung cancer	4.5	8.0
Acute upper respiratory tract infection	47.4	35.0
Acute lower respiratory tract infection	38.0	30.3
Chronic obstructive pulmonary disease	10.3	8.8
Asthma	15.2	9.6
Pulmonary embolism	1.2	1.1
Pulmonary oedema	0.2	0.2
Mitral stenosis	0.2	0.1
Bleeding disorders	0.3	0.4
Tuberculosis	0.3	0.5
Aspergillosis	0.0	0.1
Bronchiectasis	2.4	1.6

TABLE 9.3 Diagnoses at three years after presentation with rectal bleeding in general practice

Diagnosis at three years	Women (% of diagnoses)	Men (% of diagnoses)
Colorectal cancer	2.1	2.7
Peptic ulcer	1.3	1.8
Diverticulitis	7.1	5.6
Anal fissure	3.4	2.8
Crohn's disease	1.0	0.8
Ulcerative colitis	1.9	2.2
Infective colitis	4.2	3.1
Haemorrhoids	16.8	19.0
Bleeding disorders	0.4	0.2
Angiodysplasia	0.0	0.1

Thus, although the positive predictive value of rectal bleeding for colorectal cancer in men is 2.7% it is also critical to appreciate that the figure for inflammatory bowel disease (either Crohn's and Ulcerative colitis) is 3.0%. Similarly, in patients presenting with haemoptysis, it is very important to not adopt a blinkered approach and fail to consider conditions such as chronic obstructive pulmonary disease, tuberculosis or pulmonary embolism.

Recently, I encountered an individual with new onset and rapidly worsening ataxia. In this situation there are a range of diagnostic possibilities and cancer was not at the top of my list. However, the only way I could ensure that he was assessed rapidly was to 'shoehorn' him into the UK Department of Health's 'two-week wait' cancer system (which, unfortunately, added further to his anxiety). Primary care diagnostics is about ensuring that any future rapid referral systems for general practitioners be designed from the perspective of the patient with a symptom as opposed to the consultant with a special interest.

USING CLINICAL INFORMATION WISELY

Much cancer referral guidance designed for general practitioners lists, in traditional 'textbook' fashion, the symptoms and signs of the most common cancers. Unfortunately, very little consideration is often given to the applicability, the validity and the reliability of such information.

As discussed in Chapters 3 and 4, when enquiring about symptoms, these must be considered in the context of an individual's psychological, physical and cognitive state. Patients vary in their ability to recall symptoms; some may fabricate symptoms and others have a tendency to combine separate, similar symptoms into a single generic event (this tendency is referred to as telescoping).[7] Within primary care, conditions will often be encountered at an evolutionary stage when the characteristics of symptoms are changing. By the time the patient reaches the specialist clinic the description of the symptom may have become more fixed and, moreover, the patient will have had additional time to reflect on his or her story (*see also* Chapter 3, Figure 3.2: The Symptom Pyramid). To compound matters further, patients, GPs and specialists will differ in their interpretation of some common symptom terms, such as diarrhoea, constipation and heartburn.

In using clinical information from the medical history wisely I do have some particular concerns about the NICE Referral Guideline for suspected colorectal cancer that states:

1 *In patients aged 60 years and older, with rectal bleeding persisting for 6 weeks or more without a change in bowel habit and without anal symptoms, an urgent referral should be made.*

2 *In patients aged 40 years and older, reporting rectal bleeding with a change of bowel habit towards looser stools and/or increased stool frequency persisting for 6 weeks or more, an urgent referral should be made.*

3 *In patients aged 60 years and older, with a change in bowel habit to looser stools and/or more frequent stools persisting for 6 weeks or more without rectal bleeding, an urgent referral should be made.*

The published evidence certainly indicates that, in relation to the diagnosis of colorectal cancer, rectal bleeding provides a positive likelihood ratio of 10.[8] Moreover, provided that the patient actually looks at their motions (and does not have defective vision), rectal bleeding is a reliable (reproducible) symptom with a kappa value of 0.85.[9]

However, although 19% of patients within general practice will report rectal bleeding in the previous year, it is estimated that 97% of patients consulting with this symptom will not have cancer.[10,11] Therefore, it is often proposed that the medical community establish a list of features that, when observed in combination with rectal bleeding, are particularly strong indicators of colorectal cancer. These include age, specific characteristics of the bleeding, and other symptoms (both present and absent).

(a) Age:

The positive predictive values of rectal bleeding for colorectal cancer, stratified by age are shown in Table 9.4.[12]

TABLE 9.4 Age and colorectal cancer

Age group (years)	Positive predictive value
< 50	0.7
50–59	1.7
60–69	11.2
70–79	21.2

(b) Bleeding characteristics:

Traditionally it has been suggested that the risk of colorectal cancer is greater in those with new onset rectal bleeding. However a study by Norreland and Norreland indicates that similar importance should be attached to a change in a known bleeding pattern.[13]

It has also been argued that blood mixed with the stool is more suggestive of cancer than is blood coating the stool, and that dark blood mixed with stool is particularly serious. In a systematic review, finding 'blood mixed with the stool' provided a positive likelihood ratio of 1.91 and 'dark red blood' a positive likelihood ratio of 1.37, but neither of these achieved statistical significance (at the 5% level).[14]

(c) Additional symptoms:

In their recent overview, Olde Bekkink and colleagues focused on the additional discriminant value of other symptoms in patients with rectal bleeding (*see* Table 9.5).[14]

From this it seems that the presence of additional symptoms (except, perhaps, weight loss) in patients presenting with rectal bleeding are of little value in stratifying risk. The difficulties inherent in the phrase 'change in bowel habit' in terms of reliability have also been discussed previously (*see* Chapter 4).

To compound matters further, there is no data suggesting that the length of the bleeding history (i.e. 6 weeks as detailed in the NICE guidance) has any predictive value; moreover, this also ignores the frequent phenomenon of 'telescoping'[7] (*see* Chapter 4). Consequently there seems to be something slightly bewildering about setting up a rapid 'two-week referral pathway' which can only be accessed after a patient has experienced at least six weeks of bleeding! There is also evidence that, in improving survival rates of colorectal cancer patients, rectal bleeding as an initial symptom is associated with less advanced staging and reduced mortality.[15]

My personal view in relation to rectal bleeding (new onset or changed) is that, over the age of 45 years, investigation of the bowel should be offered to all patients

TABLE 9.5 Additional symptoms, rectal bleeding and colorectal cancer

Additional Symptoms	*Pooled positive likelihood ratios*
Weight loss	1.89*
Abdominal pain	0.94
Change in bowel habit	1.92
Perianal symptoms – itch/eczema	1.31
Perianal symptoms – pain on defaecation	0.49*
Previous history of rectal bleeding	0.58

*= significant result at 5% level

as soon as possible, whether or not they have other symptoms; this is an opinion shared by others working in primary care.[16] Moreover, Helford argues that the entire colon should be visualised in such individuals.[17]

One recent piece of cost-effectiveness analysis also provides some food for thought in relation to the assessment of rectal bleeding in younger people. Lewis and colleagues have concluded that the evaluation of the colon in persons 25 to 45 years of age with otherwise asymptomatic rectal bleeding increases the life expectancy at a cost comparable to that of colon cancer screening.[18]

Other symptoms that might indicate colorectal cancer (such as abdominal pain) are, unfortunately, not even considered by the NICE guidance. However, in an Exeter-based case-control study abdominal pain provided a positive likelihood ratio of 4.5 and it is suggested that the risk of colorectal cancer is increased in patients consulting with abdominal pain on at least two occasions during a six-month period.[8,19] Furthermore, in order to improve outcomes it is also worth recalling that abdominal pain is the symptom most likely to be associated with an emergency presentation, with an odds ratio of 6.2.[5]

FOCUSING ON OUTCOMES

Diagnosis is not just about detecting or excluding disease but also about considering the potential impact on patient and health service outcomes. Thus, in relation to cancer, there is a requirement for a much greater focus on what we are actually trying to achieve — the diagnosis of all cancers, or the concentration of our effort on diagnosing cancers at an earlier stage; the latter enhances the chances of cure and minimises the need for distressing and disabling, extensive and aggressive treatment. There are arguments in favour of trying to diagnose all cancers earlier; however, if we wish to improve survival then our focus ought to be on cancer identification at the earliest possible stage. Consequently, we need to push earlier symptomatic diagnosis back until it is able to be especially sensitive to the initial symptoms of a cancer rather than all the symptoms of a cancer.

One of the particular weaknesses of the NICE *Referral Guidelines for Suspected Cancer* is its imprecision in relation to diagnostic impact. There are four areas that require clarification:

(a) Which symptoms (or symptom combinations) might reflect earlier stage cancers with potential impacts on mortality, thereby improving prognosis?

(b) Which symptoms (or symptom combinations) might reflect earlier stage cancers and have a potential impact on morbidity (both from the disease and from the treatments required)?

(c) Which symptoms (or symptom combinations) might indicate already established aggressive disease that is likely to be beyond curative treatment but requires early access to palliative care?

(d) Which patients/presentations would be better served by observation over a period of time in accordance with the principles outlined in Chapter 3, i.e. ensuring that the benefits of delay (in terms of the risks of false positive diagnoses or
the avoidance of unnecessary investigations) have been carefully evaluated in
relation to the harms of delayed or missed cancer diagnoses?

As mentioned in the previous sub-section, in improving the survival from colorectal cancer it seems that rectal bleeding as an initial symptom is associated with
less advanced staging; by that logic, it warrants greater emphasis than suggested
by the current guidance.[15] For similar reasons, the possibility of colorectal cancer should be considered in all patients with iron-deficiency anaemia (not just
in men with a haemoglobin of 11 g/100 mL or less or women with a haemoglobin of 10 g/100 mL or less as suggested by NICE). For example, in a study of
431 patients in primary care with iron-deficiency anaemia (haemoglobin below
12 g/dL in males and 11 g/dL in females, with microcytosis), 7.4% of them had
colorectal cancer.[20] Moreover, some individuals in a case-control study (*see* Table
9.6) had a reduced haemoglobin result for more than a year prior to diagnosis,
perhaps representing a missed opportunity for earlier diagnosis and improved
prognosis:[21]

   At a broader level, if we continue to expect patients to consult GPs and for GPs
to initiate onward referral of such patients, in accordance with raw clinical information derived from hospital patients with established disease, it should come as no
surprise if we make little impact on the stage-specific spectrum of patients that are
seen by our hospital-based colleagues. As mentioned earlier, within primary care,
conditions will often be seen at an evolutionary stage when "text book" descrip-
tions and classifications simply do not apply. According to Mansson and colleagues,
the most common initial symptom of colorectal cancer is defecation abnormality; for breast cancer, a palpable mass in the breast; for pulmonary cancer, cough;
and for prostate cancer, symptoms of prostatism.[22] Some 'newer' features of cancers
are also now being recognised; these include impotence for prostate cancer, which
provides a positive predictive value of 3%.[23] However, as mentioned in Chapter 8,
there is an additional requirement to consider more carefully the most appropriate research design in order to identify new or novel clinical markers. For example,
only general practitioners who might be aware of a possible link between some

TABLE 9.6 Anaemia and colorectal cancer

Haemoglobin level	Positive likelihood ratio
12–12.9 g/dL	4.3
10–11.9 g/dL	3.9
< 10 g/dL	9.5

specific psychological symptoms and early pancreatic cancer[24,25] are likely to consider recording this information: a record-based case-control study of the early features of pancreatic cancer is therefore unlikely to uncover much beyond abdominal pain, weight loss and jaundice.

In Chapter 5 I also suggested that, in relation to cancer diagnosis, aside from the use of symptoms, certain pieces of clinical information more readily and uniquely available in primary care settings – such as changes in a patient's behaviour – may bear significant weight in assisting the diagnosis of malignancy. Moreover, it may even be possible to quantify such behavioural changes by looking at alterations in, perhaps, smoking status, consultation patterns (a measure of healthcare seeking behaviour), use of over-the-counter medications or accompanied surgery attendances.

Just over ten years ago I wrote to the leading authority on clinical epidemiology, Alvan R Feinstein, suggesting that what was really required to sort out cancer diagnosis was a large prospective study of symptoms, symptom combinations and other features of possible oncological significance. His response was as follows: "I think your study would be much more valuable, particularly in primary care, if you determined the frequency of explanations (diagnostic or otherwise) for the symptoms, rather than their unique or distinctive role in detecting cancers".[26] This serves as a salutary reminder that, even in undertaking research into potential cancer symptoms within primary care, it is very important to retain a broad approach.

ADOPTING A PATIENT-CENTRED APPROACH

Recently I encountered a 70-year-old gentleman with iron-deficiency anaemia and abdominal discomfort. During the course of the subsequent consultation he stated, 'Well at least one thing is certain: I don't have bowel cancer, as I had the screening test last month'. After further discussion he finally agreed to a referral – and subsequently underwent resection for his tumour. Other individuals who are non-smokers or ex-smokers have been equally bemused that I might consider them to be at risk of lung cancer.

As discussed earlier there is a lot of confusion amongst patients (and some doctors!) about disease prevention, both primary prevention and screening. This seems to be a particular problem in relation to cancer and, nowadays, in some of my discussions with patients I try to introduce the concept of cancer risk (as a user-friendly mechanism to link together Bayes' Theorem and decision-making thresholds – *see* Chapter 3) combined with seeking to explore and understand the patient's own values and concerns.

Assessing an individual's cancer risk involves a carefully-focused analysis of a patient's symptoms, family history, lifestyle and past medical history in relation to their age and sex and, if appropriate, a clinical examination and specific investigations. This process is further facilitated by the application of a number of

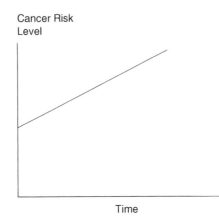

FIGURE 9.1 Cancer risk over time

computerised risk assessment tools applicable to primary care such as the OPERA tool developed for ovarian cancer risk.[27]

In relation to colorectal cancer, for example, a person can be considered to be at a certain level of individual cancer risk. As illustrated in Figure 9.1 this risk will gradually increase over time as the patient ages. On occasions the whole line might shift upwards depending on additional factors that affect the baseline risk; these may include a new medical problem (e.g. ulcerative colitis), a change in the family history or a fresh symptom (*see* Table 9.7).

Furthermore, addressing risk is about providing the patient with an evidence-based risk-reduction plan incorporating lifestyle recommendations (e.g. diet, exercise, alcohol and smoking), specific suggestions about screening (types and frequencies) and when to seek further medical attention for investigation, referral or treatment. The risk-reduction plan must be built on the risk assessment and carefully tailored to the individual as, for example, the screening plan suggested to

TABLE 9.7 Some factors influencing baseline cancer risk

Cancer Type	Some factors influencing baseline risk
Colorectal	• Family History (↑) • Personal history of Crohn's, ulcerative colitis, colorectal cancer or adenomas (↑) • Type 2 diabetes (↑)
Breast	• Hormone replacement therapy (↑) • Personal history of breast cancer, palpable cysts, atypical hyperplasia (↑) • Nulliparity, late pregnancy, early menarche, late menopause (↑) • Breastfeeding (↓)
Ovarian	• Family history (↑) • Increasing parity, early menopause, combined oral contraceptive use (↓)

(↑) = risk increase, (↓) = risk decrease

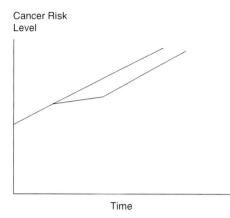

FIGURE 9.2 The impact of primary prevention activities on cancer risk

a person at elevated risk due to a family history of colorectal cancer or a history of adenomatous polyps will be different to that suggested to an asymptomatic patient whose only risk factor is being 60 years old.

Successful compliance with advice on, for example, smoking, diet or exercise (primary prevention) should result in a move down towards a new level of risk (*see* Figure 9.2).

In relation to screening it is suggested that, after an initial reduction following the screen (this reduction is related to the sensitivity of the screening test), there will be a gradual drift up towards the previous risk level; this will depend on the natural history and the incidence of the cancer. A subsequent screen will reduce the risk again, resulting in a 'saw-tooth' type risk profile (*see* Figure 9.3).

By adopting such a risk-oriented approach I would argue that it is easier to emphasise to the patient that, although such a package might reduce an individual's risk, it can *never* eliminate their risk and they should remain alert for any new

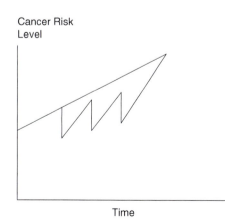

FIGURE 9.3 The impact of screening activities on cancer risk

symptoms or signs. From my perspective, the benefits of a risk-oriented approach are a better informed patient and a more balanced and focused discussion about what might (or might not) be done next.

THE APPROPRIATE USE OF INVESTIGATIONS

As emphasised in Chapter 3 the decisions made in general practice are dissimilar from those made in specialist settings — the precise diagnostic labels are often less important than deciding on an appropriate course of action. In primary care, diagnoses may be framed in terms of dichotomous decisions: treatment versus non-treatment, referral versus non-referral, and serious versus non-serious.

In this context I would therefore argue that there is a particular requirement to guard against the drift towards 'dubious precision', with inappropriate testing leading to unwarranted delays or unnecessary additional service costs. By considering the diagnostic processing pathway it is clear that, after the patient has furnished the GP with a medical history, the decision-making threshold for onward referral might already have been exceeded such that even a relatively simple investigation will have no further impact on this referral decision.

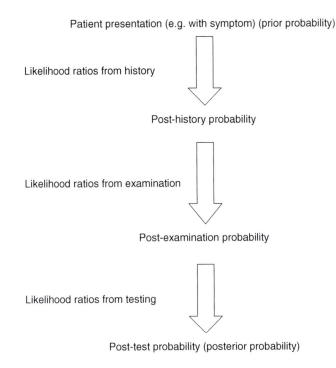

Patient presentation (e.g. with symptom) (prior probability)

Likelihood ratios from history

Post-history probability

Likelihood ratios from examination

Post-examination probability

Likelihood ratios from testing

Post-test probability (posterior probability)

For example, according to Leicester and colleagues, haemoccult has a high specificity for colorectal cancer in symptomatic patients (84.5%).[28] Thus, in accord with the rule of SpPin (*see* Chapter 3: 'if a test has sufficiently high specificity, a positive result rules in the disorder'), haemoccult testing may be useful in adding further evidence to a diagnostic problem. However, in view of the lower sensitivity (the haemoccult test fails to detect 20–50% of cancers and up to 80% of polyps), a negative result cannot be used in symptomatic patients to rule out colorectal cancer. I was therefore somewhat bewildered recently to encounter a patient with rectal bleeding who had been given a series of faecal occult blood tests with a subsequent delay of at least a further four weeks before onward referral!

For my part, I have often wondered whether it is worthwhile undertaking a full blood count in patients with rectal bleeding. Anaemia certainly increases the risk (i.e. Hb <12 g/100 mL for women or <13.3 g/100 mL for men provides a positive likelihood ratio of 3.67 for colorectal cancer diagnosis) but – as I will already have made a decision to refer a patient for further investigations based on the presence of rectal bleeding – the result of the blood count will not impact on my decision. Others might consider that the 'absence of anaemia' reduces the risk, but from the paper by Olde Bekkink *et al.* it is possible to calculate a negative likelihood ratio of 0.87 for anaemia, which is insufficient to argue against a diagnosis of colorectal cancer.[14] So it is important that any additional investigations such as a full blood count (that certainly might be of assistance to our hospital-based specialist colleagues) do not produce any delay in initiating an onward referral in a patient with rectal bleeding.

One particular difficulty that always needs to be borne in mind is that, within primary care settings, the vast majority of symptoms seem to defy a clear-cut, organic explanation. As mentioned in Chapter 2, Kroenke and Mangelsdorff demonstrated that no specific physical disorder could be established as the cause in 30–75% of instances, even after careful investigation.[29] Obviously, it is always necessary to exclude organic disease when presented with a symptom of possible oncological significance, but there is also a requirement to avoid undertaking investigations beyond those that are absolutely necessary.

In recent years I have become particularly concerned that worry of 'missing' cancers is leading to the over-investigation of some non-specific symptoms by GPs; this carries the potential for adverse impacts on patient wellbeing, as well as on the overall healthcare budget. More specifically I would suggest that, in patients presenting with fatigue/tiredness, too many pathology tests are undertaken too early in the course of the symptom, often with inadequate consideration of other factors from the medical history and the physical examination. Fatigue is the second most common symptom presenting to general practitioners (lifetime prevalence of 23.6%)[30] and, in 2008, Harrison pointed out that general practitioners investigated between 56% and 62% of all tired patients compared with 11% in 2004.[31] Furthermore, the number of tests/test groups ordered has increased from three to nearly four since 2004. An additional problem is the 'cascade' effect of mildly abnormal results generating further tests across all of the diagnostic domains (especially imaging, endoscopy and pathology). Certainly, as the prior probability of underlying somatic pathology may be expected to be less than 5% in unselected patients, the likelihood of false-positive results is very high. Interestingly other work has demonstrated that, after two weeks' follow-up, 58% of such patients presenting will have improved.[32]

Looking to the published literature for some guidance it seems that in an audit of 181 patients investigated for tiredness, only 3% had a significant clinical diagnosis based on an abnormal pathology result.[33] In Norway, Mansson *et al.* also noted the considerable expense of seeking to investigate some symptoms of possible oncological significance in the community.[34] More specifically tiredness/fatigue had particularly high investigation costs but detected no cases of cancer in their study.

One way forward might be to consider 'delayed testing'. In a recently completed PhD study of blood test ordering for unexplained fatigue in general practice[35] it was noted (by means of a randomised controlled trial) that a watchful waiting approach (as opposed to an immediate testing approach) reduced mean costs of testing from €215.83 per patient to €151.34 with no other adverse impacts on referrals or outcomes.

Currently it is being argued that GPs should have enhanced direct access to more complex radiology in order for us to improve our ability to diagnose abdominal or thoracic malignancies. Although this proposal might steal some headlines, I do have some doubts about whether it is really appropriate for me to have unfettered access to computed tomography (CT) scans for my patients with abdominal or chest symptoms. Aside from the risks of excessive radiation exposure, the published evidence is not supportive of such a blanket approach. For example, Master and colleagues studied 137 patients with non-acute abdominal pain referred for computed tomography by U.S. family practitioners and concluded that the majority received no diagnosis and, moreover, that CT was rarely diagnostic for patients lacking a warning feature.[36] Of further concern, positive and unrelated CT findings were equally prevalent and the latter were not beneficial to patients. In a separate audit of the use of thoracic computed tomography by general practitioners in Cairns it was concluded that many CT examinations of the chest requested by GPs could be avoided or replaced by simpler, cheaper tests with lower radiation exposure.[37] Moreover, it was estimated that the radiation exposure involved in these unnecessary chest CT scans could be responsible for about 40 fatal cancers per year in Australia.

However there is a balance to be struck as it has also been suggested that some general practitioners might be overly resistant to the use of investigations in patients presenting with subjective symptoms such as non-acute abdominal/pelvic discomfort, possibly contributing to the adverse outcomes for individuals with ovarian or pancreatic malignancies.

When faced with a patient complaining of non-acute abdominal/pelvic discomfort a range of options might be available to the general practitioner seeking to rule out significant conditions such as malignancy (in addition to ruling in conditions such as ureteric calculi): i.e. abdominal ultrasound, pelvic ultrasound, trans-vaginal ultrasound, CT scanning or MRI, acute referral, chronic referral, alternative investigations, and 'watchful waiting'. The difficulty is to determine the most appropriate next step from this range of nine possibilities, given that some pose more risks to patients than others.

Building on the work by myself and my colleagues in relation to the appropriate use of BNP/Echo for heart failure (*see* Chapter 10), appropriateness ratings should soon be generated for the investigation of some of the commoner subjective symptoms of possible oncological significance such as non-acute abdominal/pelvic discomfort and headache.

CONCLUSION

Seeking to make a diagnosis of possible cancer in primary care can be perplexing; it is particularly complicated if GPs choose to ignore their surroundings. Symptoms are not synonymous with organic disease, nor is primary care medicine merely a faded memory of hospital-based practice. In seeking to make a diagnostic decision when faced with a symptom of 'possible oncological significance', it is particularly necessary to consider matters in the context of primary care and from the perspective of the patient.

GENERAL REFERENCES

- Hamilton WT, Peters TJ, editors. *Cancer Diagnosis in Primary Care*. Elsevier: London, 2007.
- National Institute for Health and Clinical Excellence. *Referral Guidelines for Suspected Cancer*. NICE: London, 2005.
- Summerton N. *Diagnosing Cancer in Primary Care*. Radcliffe: Oxford, 1999.

TEXT REFERENCES

1. Love N. Why patients delay seeking care for cancer symptoms. What you can do about it. *Postgraduate Medicine* 1991; 89: 151–8.
2. Robinson M, Thomas W, Hardcastle JD, *et al*. Change towards earlier stage at presentation of colorectal cancer. *Brit J Surg* 1993; 80: 1610–12.
3. Gatta G, Cappocaccia R, Sant M, *et al*. Understanding variations in survival for colorectal cancer in Europe: a EUROCARE high resolution study. *Gut* 2000; 47: 533–8.
4. Hargarten SW, Roberts MJS, Anderson AJ. Cancer presentation in the emergency department: a failure of primary care. *Am J Emerg Med* 1992; 10: 290–3.
5. Cleary J, Peters TJ, Sharp D, Hamilton W. Clinical features of colorectal cancer before emergency presentation: a population-based case-control study. *Family Practice* 2007; 24: 3–6.

6. Jones R, Charlton J, Latinovic R, Gulliford MC. Alarm symptoms and identification of non-cancer diagnoses in primary care: cohort study. *BMJ* 2009; **339**: 491–3.

7. Barsky AJ. Forgetting, fabricating and telescoping. The instability of the medical history. *Arch Intern Med* 2002; **162**: 981–4.

8. Hamilton W, Round A, Sharp D, Peters TJ. Clinical features of colorectal cancer before diagnosis: a population-based case-control study. *B J Cancer* 2005; **93**: 399–405.

9. Summerton N, Mann S, Sutton J, *et al*. Developing clinically relevant and reproducible symptom-defined populations for cancer diagnostic research in general practice using a community survey. *Family Practice* 2003; **20**: 340–6.

10. Crosland A, Jones R. Rectal bleeding: prevalence and consultation behaviour. *BMJ* 1995; **311**: 486–8.

11. Robertson R, Campbell C, Weller DP, *et al*. Predicting colorectal cancer risk in patients with rectal bleeding. *Brit J General Practice* 2006; **56**: 763–7.

12. Waters H, Casteren VV, Buntinx F. Rectal bleeding and colorectal cancer in general practice: diagnostic study. *BMJ* 2000; **321**: 998–9.

13. Norrelund N, Norrelund H. Colorectal cancer and polyps in patients aged 40 years and over who consult a GP with rectal bleeding. *Family Practice* 1996; **13**: 160–5.

14. Olde Bekkink M, McCowan C, Falk GA, *et al*. Diagnostic accuracy systematic review of rectal bleeding in combination with other symptoms, signs and tests in relation to colorectal cancer. *B J Cancer* 2010; **102**: 48–58.

15. Stapley S, Peters TJ, Sharp D, Hamilton W. The mortality of colorectal cancer in relation to the initial symptom at presentation to primary care and to the duration of symptoms: a cohort study using medical records. *B J Cancer* 2006; **95**: 1321–5.

16. Du Toit J, Hamilton W, Barraclough K. Risk in primary care of colorectal cancer from new onset rectal bleeding: 10 year prospective study. *BMJ* 2006; **333**: 69–70.

17. Helfand M, Marton KI, Zimmer-Gembeck M, Sox HC. History of visible rectal bleeding in a primary care population. Initial assessment and 10-year follow-up. *JAMA* 1997; **277**: 44–8.

18. Lewis JD, Brown A, Localio R, Schwartz JS. Initial evaluation of rectal bleeding in young persons: a cost-effectiveness analysis. *Ann Intern Med* 2002; **136**: 99–110.

19. Hamilton WT. Derivation of a score for identifying colorectal cancer in primary care. *Gut* 2007; **56**(Suppl. 2): A49.

20. Logan E, Yates J, Stewart R, *et al*. Investigation and management of iron deficiency anaemia in general practice. *Postgrad Med J* 2002; **78**: 533–7.

21. Hamilton W, Lancashire R, Sharp D, *et al*. The importance of anaemia in diagnosing colorectal cancer: a case-control study using electronic primary care records. *Brit J Cancer* 2008; **98**: 323–7.

22. Mansson J, Björkelund C, Hultborn R. Symptom pattern and diagnostic work-up of malignancy at first symptom presentation as related to level of care. A retrospective study from the primary healthcare centre area of Kungsbacka, Sweden. *Neoplasma* 1999; **46**: 93–9.

23. Hamilton W, Sharp D, Peters TJ, Round A. Clinical features of prostate cancer before diagnosis: a population-based case-control study. *Brit J Gen Pract* 2006; **56**: 756–82.

24. Yaskin J. Nervous symptoms as early manifestations of carcinoma of the pancreas. *JAMA* 1931; **96**: 1664–8.

25. Passik SD, Roth AJ. Anxiety symptoms and panic attacks preceding pancreatic cancer diagnosis. *Psycho-oncology* 1999; **8**: 268–72.

26. Summerton, N. Conversation with: Feinstein AR. 2000 July 17.

27. www.macmillan.org.uk/Aboutus/Healthprofessionals/Cancer genetics/OPERA. aspx (accessed 10 December 2010).

28. Leicester RJ, Lightfoot A, Millar J, *et al.* Accuracy and value of the Hemoccult test in symptomatic patients. *BMJ* 1983; **286**: 673–4.

29. Kroenke K, Mangelsdorff D. Common symptoms in ambulatory care. *Am J Med* 1989; **86**: 262–6.

30. Kroenke K, Price RK. Symptoms in the community. Prevalance, classification and psychiatric comorbidity. *Arch Intern Med* 1993; **153**: 2474–80.

31. Harrison M. Pathology testing in the tired patient. A rational approach. *Australian Family Physician* 2008; **37**: 908–10.

32. Kroenke K, Jackson JL. Outcome in general medical patients presenting with common symptoms: a prospective study with a 2-week and a 3-month follow-up. *Family Practice* 1998; **15**: 398–403.

33. Gialamas A, Beilby JJ, Pratt NL, *et al.* Investigating tiredness in Australian general practice. Do pathology tests help in diagnosis? *Australian Family Physician* 2003; **32**: 663–6.

34. Mansson J, Marklund B, Carlsson P. Costs in primary care of investigating symptoms suspicious of cancer in a defined population. *Scand J Prim Health Care* 2006; **24**: 243–50.

35. Van Bokhoven L. *Blood test ordering for unexplained complaints in general practice. The feasibility of a watchful waiting approach.* University of Maastricht: Maastricht, 2008.

36. Master SS, Longstreth GF, Liu AL. Results of computed tomography in family practitioners' patients with non-acute abdominal pain. *Family Practice* 2005; **22**: 474–7.

37. Simpson G, Hartrick GS. Use of thoracic computed tomography by general practitioners. *Medical Journal of Australia* 2007; **187**: 43–6.

CHAPTER 10

The application of primary care diagnostics 2: commissioning

The commissioning of diagnostic services directly accessible from primary care has always been somewhat haphazard, often driven more by local specialist clinical interests or technological innovations than the needs of patients. For example, as a GP working in East Yorkshire I have unfettered access to BNP testing, yet cannot order an MRI scan for any individual with back problems. By contrast, my colleagues just across the Pennines can arrange CT scans with alacrity but BNP testing remains unavailable to them.

In seeking to commission diagnostic services, one particular difficulty arises from the categorisation of diagnostics into four separate domains: endoscopy, imaging, pathology and physiological testing. Within the UK, the Department of Health has re-emphasised these divisions by the appointment of four national clinical leads. To confound matters further, although the National Institute for Health and Clinical Excellence (NICE) is charged with appraising diagnostic technologies to assist commissioners, its remit is restricted to new technologies.

For primary care clinicians the current siloed approach makes no sense; moreover, the most powerful diagnostic technology – the medical history – has largely been ignored by most policymakers. For example, in seeking to diagnose an individual with cardio-respiratory symptoms (e.g. dyspnoea, cough, haemoptysis, palpitations or chest pain) I might require access to one or more of the following tests after taking a history and examining the patient: spirometry, oximetry, electrocardiography, echocardiography, imaging, endoscopy, BNP testing, biochemistry, haematology or sputum microscopy. Similarly, in individuals with ENT symptoms (e.g. deafness, earache/discharge, tinnitus, hoarseness or nasal symptoms), I might subsequently need to arrange audiometry, tympanometry, imaging, microbiology, haematology, allergy testing or indirect laryngoscopy.

The emphasis on hospital-based testing services has also allowed some concerns expressed about the quality of diagnostic technologies directly delivered within primary care to remain unaddressed. It now seems that anyone is permitted to take a medical history; there is no requirement for specific training to understand the complexities of symptom reporting, symptom evolution, symptom classification or symptom interpretation as discussed in Chapter 4. In relation to near-patient biochemistry testing within general practice, there can be quite marked variations from the true values.[1] More recently, others have worried about ECG interpretation by general practitioners and the delivery of spirometry services within primary care.[2,3] According to the Department of Health's National Imaging Board[4] the uncontrolled expansion of the use of ultrasound represents a significant current clinical risk if:

- examinations are undertaken by untrained or poorly trained individuals
- equipment is poorly specified or poorly maintained
- it is undertaken in the absence of a clinical audit of performance

As increasing numbers of investigations are delivered in community settings, issues of clinical governance will require a much greater focus. It is therefore very important to ensure that any drive towards enhanced test accessibility does not take precedence over issues of quality and safety.

Even if a decision is made by a general practitioner to arrange an 'open access' or 'near-patient' test, the question of exactly when to test also needs to be carefully considered. There is a wealth of evidence indicating that many tests are repeated unnecessarily[5] and, in the case of monitoring, undertaken too early with a risk that the 'signal' becomes lost in the 'noise'.[6] There is also an ongoing debate about whether general practitioners make 'appropriate' use of a particular diagnostic service. As illustrated in Chapter 2 many specialists take the view that they are the ultimate arbiters of the appropriateness of GP actions, whereas I prefer a more 'primary care-based' approach, one based on the ideas developed in this book. It is also important to appreciate that appropriateness includes not only overuse or misuse of diagnostic techniques, but should also consider underuse.

A further consideration is whether a specific test is the best approach in comparison with alternative investigations (across all testing domains) and strategies. For example in some patients presenting with cardio-respiratory symptoms the evidence suggests that B-type natriuretic peptide (BNP) might be used as a 'rule out' triage test prior to echocardiography whereas others should progress directly to echocardiography without an intervening stage.[7] In patients with probable transient ischaemic attacks (TIAs), an alternative to 'open access' carotid ultrasound is a "TIA clinic" that offers the patient a range of investigations together with a rapid specialist opinion.[8]

In recent years I have been fortunate enough to have been given the opportunity to apply the principles of primary care diagnostics to work I have undertaken with colleagues in London and Cumbria. In this chapter I shall outline two specific outcomes of this programme of work that might be of assistance to others seeking to adopt a more systematic approach to the commissioning of direct access diagnostic services: assessing needs and developing services, and rating appropriateness.

ASSESSING NEEDS AND DEVELOPING SERVICES

Diagnosis is not just about detecting or excluding disease, but also about considering the potential impact of a particular pathway on patient and health service outcomes. In most circumstances, diagnosis involves a sequence of tests rather than a single investigation and consideration should be given to inputs (e.g. new onset dyspnoea) and outputs (e.g. the diagnosis of heart failure, death from cancer or disability from rheumatoid arthritis) in addition to specific tests. It is now suggested that a good mechanism to link these three elements and thereby identify diagnostic testing needs and commission services is by identifying and populating symptom-initiated diagnostic processing pathways (SiDPPs) based on the following sequence (*see* Chapter 3):

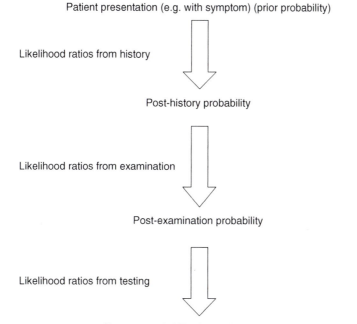

SiDPPs make clinical sense and also encourage balanced, rational and forward-looking commissioning. They can facilitate improvements in overall diagnostic efficiency and effectiveness with benefits for individual patient care as well as the healthcare budget. Moreover, when diagnosis is viewed as a processing pathway founded on a robust medical history, it becomes clear that in some situations investigations may become unnecessary and, in other circumstances, their impact will be enhanced. Conversely, if diagnostic testing is not considered in the context of a diagnostic processing pathway there is an increased risk that investigations may be used inappropriately with a higher chance of false positives in a lower prevalence population.

From the commissioner's perspective it is also important to be aware that diagnosis is not the only reason for which a test might be ordered. For that reason, consideration also needs to be given to the other potential purposes of a test: screening, monitoring, risk/treatment stratification and prognostic assessment.

Aims

There are three overarching aims of any direct access diagnostic needs assessment (and subsequent service developments):

1 **Impacting on test provision.** This is about developing a menu of tests that might be considered for direct access by primary care clinicians. However, in addition, both pre-testing requirements and test support (such as education, training, infrastructure and quality assurance) must be considered in order to ensure that the potential benefits of a test are realised.

2 **Enhancing the quality of diagnostic processing, monitoring, risk/treatment stratification, screening and prognostic assessment.** This is about addressing the following:

- clinical effectiveness, which incorporates appropriateness and efficiency
- patient-centredness covering accessibility (time, place and person), acceptability and timeliness. Equity is considered within both accessibility and acceptability.
- safety

3 **Improving patient and health service outcomes.** This over laps with 2 but, in relation to diagnosis, is primarily about seeking to:

- minimise the number of diagnoses completely missed and their related adverse impacts on mortality, morbidity, and patient satisfaction
- minimise the number of delayed diagnoses that, in turn, retard appropriate therapeutic interventions and have negative effects on mortality, morbidity, and patient satisfaction
- minimise the number of incorrect diagnoses that may lead to inappropriate or even harmful treatment, physical and psychological morbidity, patient dissatisfaction/discomfort and unnecessary expenditure
- minimise the inappropriate or excessive use of diagnostic tests or procedures beyond those needed to make a diagnosis in a timely and cost-effective manner. Test overuse can lead to physical and psychological morbidity and patient dissatisfaction/discomfort. Clearly, this issue is also particularly relevant to the use of tests as disease monitoring tools.

Approach

In appreciation of the principles of primary care diagnostics outlined in this book, the following approach to examining directly-accessible diagnostic/testing needs is suggested:

Diagnostic testing

This should be assessed by identifying and populating ten broadly-defined symptom-initiated diagnostic processing pathways (SiDPPs):

1 cardio-respiratory symptoms
2 abdominal symptoms

3 neck/back symptoms
4 headache and facial pain/swelling
5 joint and limb symptoms
6 transient alterations of consciousness
7 skin, hair and nail symptoms
8 urinary and testicular symptoms
9 pelvic and menstrual symptoms
10 ENT symptoms

Non-diagnostic testing

Consideration also needs to be given to the other potential purposes of a test (i.e. screening, monitoring, risk/treatment stratification and prognostic assessment) by developing condition-specific matrices, for instance:

• colorectal and prostate cancers (screening, stratification and monitoring)
• osteoporosis (screening, stratification and monitoring)
• atherosclerotic disease (screening, stratification and monitoring)
• specific chronic diseases e.g. diabetes, COPD and asthma
• therapeutic drug (and adverse event) monitoring e.g. for individuals with rheumatoid disease, heart failure, renal dysfunction, thyroid disorders, hypertension, epilepsy and for those patients on warfarin

Overarching principles

Using Tables 10.1 and 10.2 as a guide, any open access testing needs assessment should pay particular attention to the following:

Accessible

• What range of tests is currently accessible to GPs for their patients?
• Is the current testing service accessible at a convenient range of times, days and locations?
• Is the current testing accessible to all (i.e. equitable)?
• What range of tests is currently available at the same time i.e. 'one stop shop' or in specific symptom-oriented clinics?
• Is information on current tests accessible in form, content and location?

Acceptable

• Have individuals undergoing testing been provided with adequate information on the proposed test (e.g. covering issues such as purpose, accuracy, implications) in order to make an informed choice?
• Is the information on the test presented in a way that considers the individual's understanding, culture and language?
• What proportion of samples or results is currently lost, inadequate, undertaken at the wrong time or not reviewed/acted upon?

TABLE 10.1 Symptom-initiated diagnostic processing pathways (SiDPPs)

Major SiDPPs	Suggested 'open access' menu	Key conditions to consider (in relation to testing/referral by GPs)
Cardio-respiratory symptoms (Group 1): • breathlessness • chest pain • palpitations • cough • haemoptysis	• chest X-Ray • echo • ECG • exercise ECG • ambulatory ECG recording/ event recording • spirometry (with reversibility) • BNP • biochemistry and haematology • sputum microscopy, culture and sensitivity • pulse oximetry • also see group 2 • specific symptom clinics	• obstructive/restrictive lung disease • heart failure • pneumonia • ischaemic heart disease • aortic aneurysm • pulmonary conditions, e.g. pneumothorax, PE, effusion • infective conditions, e.g. pneumonia, TB, bronchiectasis • malignancy • cardiomyopathies • arrhythmias • general, e.g. diabetes, thyroid, anaemia • paediatric – foreign body, bronchiolitis, cystic fibrosis • GI reflux (see 2)
Abdominal symptoms (Group 2): • abdominal pain • abdominal swelling • change in bowel habit (diarrhoea and/or constipation) • nausea and vomiting (including blood) • rectal bleeding and discharge • jaundice • dyspepsia • dysphagia	• abdominal ultrasound • barium studies (selected) • sigmoidoscopy • urine/stool microscopy, culture and sensitivity (including blood) • colonoscopy • biochemistry and haematology • H. Pylori testing • upper GI endoscopy • coeliac testing • hepatitis serology • autoantibodies and CRP • allergy testing • specific symptom clinics	• aortic aneurysm • liver, gallbladder and pancreas dysfunction • infective conditions, e.g. bowel and bladder (adults and children) • upper GI conditions, e.g. ulceration/reflux • lower GI conditions, e.g. diverticulitis, inflammatory bowel disease, coeliac • renal dysfunction and stones • malignancy • general, e.g. diabetes, thyroid, sickling • allergies
Neck/back symptoms (Group 3): • neck/backache • neck/back stiffness	• imaging (X-ray, MRI) • ESR/CRP and plasma electrophoresis • PSA	• disc and spinal disorders (including stenosis) • fractures • aortic aneurysm

TABLE 10.1 Symptom-initiated diagnostic processing pathways (SiDPPs)

Major SiDPPs	Suggested 'open access' menu	Key conditions to consider (in relation to testing/referral by GPs)
	• specific symptom clinics • see also group 2	• urinary stones • infective conditions, e.g. osteomyelitis, UTI • malignancy
Headache and facial pain/swelling (Group 4):	• CT/MRI • ESR/CRP • sialogram/ultrasound • specific symptom clinics • haematology	• temporal arteritis • oral/dental disorders • space occupying lesion • subarachnoid haemorrhage • parotid conditions, e.g. stones/obstruction • infective conditions, e.g. meningitis, encephalitis • malignancy
Joint and limb symptoms (Group 5): • pain/aches • stiffness • paraesthesia • swelling	• imaging (X-ray, MRI) • Rh factor, CRP, autoantibodies • nerve conduction studies • microscopy, culture and sensitivity of joint fluid • uric acid • D-Dimer • Doppler studies (venous and arterial) • biochemistry and haematology • also see group 1 • specific symptom clinics	• arthritis – inflammatory, septic, osteoarthritis • knee dysfunction, e.g. meniscus • fracture • avascular necrosis • spinal disorders • neuropathies (including entrapment) • peripheral vascular disease • DVT • TIA/stroke • malignancy • polymyalgia/connective tissue diseases • paediatric –slipped epiphysis
Transient alterations of consciousness (Group 6):	• EEG plus interpretation • CT/MRI • carotid ultrasound • biochemistry and haematology • also see group 1 • specific symptom clinics	• epilepsy • arrhythmias • TIA/stroke • general, e.g. diabetes
Skin, hair and nail symptoms/signs (Group 7):	• mycology • autoantibodies • allergy testing • tele-dermatology • specific symptom clinics	• malignancy • allergies • fungal disorders

(Continued)

TABLE 10.1 Symptom-initiated diagnostic processing pathways (SiDPPs) (*Continued*)

Major SiDPPs	Suggested 'open access' menu	Key conditions to consider (in relation to testing/referral by GPs)
Urinary and testicular symptoms (Group 8): • scrotal swelling • testicular pain • haematuria • voiding or obstructive symptoms • storage or irritative symptoms	• cystoscopy • urinalysis • biochemistry and haematology • microscopy, culture and sensitivity of urine. • PSA • abdominal and pelvic ultrasound • plain X-ray of abdomen • testicular ultrasound • urine cytology • urodynamic studies • specific symptom clinics	• urinary infection and stones • urinary dysfunction (children) • testicular disorders, e.g. torsion and infection • prostate disorders and strictures • malignancy
Pelvic and menstrual symptoms (Group 9): • pain • dyspareunia • abnormal bleeding	• pelvic/vaginal ultrasound • microbiology • pregnancy testing • hormone profiles • colposcopy • endometrial sampling • haematology • specific symptom clinics	• menopause • malignancy • polycystic ovaries/cysts • endometriosis • polyps/fibroids • pelvic infections • pregnancy-related conditions (e.g. ectopic, miscarriage)
ENT symptoms (Group 10): • deafness • earache and discharge • tinnitus • hoarseness • nasal symptoms • vertigo	• pure tone audiogram • tympanometry • imaging • microbiology (throat and ear) • glandular fever tests and CRP • indirect laryngoscopy • allergy testing • also see Group 2. • specific symptom clinics	• infective conditions • malignancy

NB: Some focused problems such as eye disorders, breast lumps and forgetfulness have not been included in the table.

Efficient
- Is the turnaround time linked to the clinical requirements?
- Is there a tendency to repeat tests unnecessarily?
- Is the staffing, transport and information technology used optimised?
- Are there any disinvestment opportunities in relation to the currently available range of tests that would have no detrimental impact on cost-effective patient care?

TABLE 10.2 Condition-specific matrix of some selected 'open access' tests by other purposes

Selected examples	Monitoring	Screening	Stratification
Osteoporosis	• DEXA	• DEXA (following FRAX score)	• FRAX Score[9]
Atherosclerotic disease (including those on therapies)	• BP • lipids • biochemistry	• BP • lipids • biochemistry • abdominal aortic aneurysm screening	• ankle-brachial pressure index • carotid ultrasound • calcium Score • exercise ECG

Quality assured and safe

- Are robust clinical governance systems (including risk management, internal/external quality assurance, audit and training) in place?
- Have specific safety issues, including infection control, errors (e.g. in identification and transmission), adherence to standard operating procedures, test performance characteristics and the approach to abnormal results (tester and recipient) been considered?

Timely

- Does a specific test make any significant contribution to a SiDPP? This impact can be graded from minus five (i.e. negative contribution) through zero (no contribution) to five (maximal contribution).
- Is any aspect of the current testing process (accessing/ordering, undertaking, transporting, reporting/communicating and interpreting) a rate-limiting step, and might resulting delays in progression lead to adverse outcomes such as morbidity and mortality?

Co-ordinated and comprehensive

- Is there a co-ordinated approach with a rational balance between the high technology (e.g. CT/MRI) and lower technology (e.g. the clinical assessment, clinical prediction rules and simple biochemistry, imaging and physiological investigations) testing services?
- What are the alternatives? Any test should be considered not only against similar technologies (e.g. imaging versus imaging) but also in relation to and in conjunction with other approaches (e.g. imaging versus history/examination/prediction rules and/or versus physiological measurement and/or versus endoscopy and/or versus testing combinations, e.g. for triage).

Contextually aware

- What is the setting/population within which any test is (or might be) used?

- Is the test setting rural or urban? Remote and rural areas might have distinct testing requirements dictated by their geography, transport systems and communication infrastructure.
- Is there an appreciation of other key local and national health policy developments?
- Is there any consideration of likely trends in demographics, disease, biomedical knowledge, therapeutics and testing technologies?

Prioritisation

From the assessment of needs it is important to select some key priorities for service development. To achieve this, the following issues should be considered:

Burden of avoidable disease, disability, dissatisfaction and death

- Would a focus on this SiDPP or test purpose address issues that are associated with significant local concerns related to testing and clinical effectiveness, patient centredness and/or testing quality, and safety in the population as a whole or in particular subgroups?
- Would a focus on this SiDPP or test purpose significantly improve local patient/carer centredness, and/or address issues of ineffectiveness and/or quality and safety, and/or reduce inequalities in health relative to existing practice?
- Is a focus on this SiDPP or test purpose likely to impact on the current burden of avoidable disease (including disease stage), death, dissatisfaction, discomfort or disability locally?

Likely resource impact

- Would a focus on this SiDPP or test purpose relate to one or more interventions or practices that might impact significantly on local NHS or other societal financial resources?
- Might a focus on this SiDPP or test purpose lead to a substantive improvement in cost efficiency in the local delivery of healthcare?
- Would a focus on this SiDPP or test purpose relate to interventions from which the local NHS could disinvest without detriment to cost-effective patient care, thus freeing up resources for use elsewhere in the local NHS?

Variation in practice

- Is there significant evidence of inappropriate local practice or variation in practice across the locality in relation to the components a SiDPP or the delivery of a test purpose?
- Might a focus on this SiDPP or test purpose impact on the current levels of inappropriate testing practice or variation in testing practice?
- Is a focus on this SiDPP or test purpose likely to impact on any local variation in access to tests or subsequent treatment (between geographical areas or social groups)?

Outputs

Possible outputs from a primary care-oriented testing needs assessment might include a proposed menu of tests (types and settings) directly accessible by primary care clinicians, pre-testing requirements for primary care clinicians linked to the menu of tests, testing intelligence to support clinical practice and suggested service specifications. Any testing service specification will also need to specifically consider the following issues:

- Where should the technology be located? Possible delivery formats include near-patient testing, tele-testing, mobile testing or centralised testing with, perhaps, remote components such as phlebotomy.
- Who should deliver the testing? Is there are place for a 'multiskilled' community-based testing technician or a specific clinic?
- What is the most cost-effective, efficient, accessible, acceptable, equitable and appropriate sequence of components in the SiDPP and any monitoring/screening pathways?
- How should Bayesian processing and decision-making thresholds be used for both diagnosis and monitoring (*see* Chapter 3)? Are there circumstances in which the disease probability after the history and the examination (the post-examination probability) is such that undertaking any diagnostic investigation is actually unnecessary, regardless of its likelihood ratio?
- What should the approach be to abnormalities aside from symptoms such as signs (e.g. breast lumps) and incidental test findings (e.g. raised glucose)?
- What should the approach be to other diagnostic strategies used within primary care such as the 'test of time' for certain SiDPPs (*see* Chapter 3)?
- What should the approach be to 'new/unforeseen' abnormalities identified by a non-specific technology (incidentalomas) or disease that would never have become apparent to an individual during their lifetime had they not undergone the diagnostic test (pseudo disease)?
- How should new technologies be accommodated within an existing SiDPP? Straightforward substitution is not appropriate unless the new test detects the same spectrum or subgroup of disease as the old test, or treatment response is similar across the spectrum of disease.[10]

Practical Example: Osteoporosis and DEXA scanning

In Cumbria, my discussions with specialist colleagues and the commissioners identified DEXA scanning (linked to osteoporosis screening, stratification and monitoring) as a particular priority. This was confirmed in a more detailed questionnaire survey of local general practitioners.

Assessing needs

In order to explore the issue further, current service specifications were obtained and routine NHS data sources were examined:

Provision

In recent years, across England, there has been a gradual trend toward a reduction in DEXA waiting times. Within Cumbria, NHS commissioning data revealed that DEXA scanning was mainly provided by two hospital-based units. Furthermore, NHS waiting time data (which represents a 'snap shot' of the waiting list on the last day of a particular month) was combined with NHS activity data (which details the actual number of DEXA scans carried out in a particular month) and compared with similar data sourced from other localities. This led to the conclusion that, although there was a reasonable amount of activity across Cumbria, this activity did not meet the demand.

Accessibility

This was assessed by examining DEXA attendance by postcode, as this provided some information on the distance travelled and, moreover, whether some areas had lower utilisation than others (if so, this might be related to accessibility). More detailed work is still required to adjust this data according to population characteristics and also to clarify the sources and purposes of DEXA requests.

Impact

Clearly the purpose of DEXA scanning is to impact on the incidence of osteoporotic fractures. In order to assess this need, routinely collected NHS data was obtained on the following:

- *Emergency admissions for fractured neck of femur*
- *Hospital procedures: primary hip replacement*
- *Hospital procedures: revision hip replacement*
- *Emergency readmissions to hospital within 28 days of discharge; fractured proximal femur*
- *Returning to usual place of residence following hospital treatment: fractured proximal femur*
- *Deaths within 30 days of emergency admission to hospital: fractured proximal femur*
- *Mortality from fracture of femur*

In addition, information was sought on osteoporosis-related prescribing and on accidents.

Considering future trends

In planning any osteoporosis testing service it is also important to give some consideration to any likely changes in the population, guidelines and technologies.

Demographics In relation to future trends in the incidence and prevalence of osteoporosis, the following factors are of particular importance: age; prolonged loss of mobility; chronic diseases such as coeliac, liver disease, renal dysfunction and rheumatoid arthritis; current smoking habits; and excessive alcohol intake.[11] In Cumbria, the rapidly ageing population presents a particular challenge for osteoporosis-related services.

Guidelines In recent years it has become apparent that the presence of several of the risk factors used to trigger a DEXA scan is associated with a fracture risk greater than can be accounted for by bone mineral density (BMD) alone. Thus, it has been suggested that the assessment of fracture risk take account of those clinical risk factors that contribute to fracture risk in addition to BMD, since this increases the detection rate of individuals prone to fracture. The FRAX tool for the assessment of fracture risk[9] integrates clinical risk factors, with or without femoral neck BMD, to calculate the 10-year probability of a major osteoporotic fracture (spine, hip, forearm or proximal humerus).

Therefore it is now suggested that:

- postmenopausal women with a prior fragility fracture be considered for treatment without the need for further risk assessment, although BMD measurement may sometimes be appropriate, particularly in younger postmenopausal women
- assessment by the FRAX tool be undertaken in:
  - men aged 50 years or more (with or without fracture) but with a WHO risk factor or a BMI < 19 kg/m²
  - all postmenopausal women without fracture but with a WHO risk factor or a BMI < 19 kg/m²
- following the assessment of fracture risk using FRAX, the patient may be classified as low, intermediate or high risk with the following possible advice:
  - low risk – reassure and reassess in 5 years or less depending on the clinical context.
  - intermediate risk – measure BMD and recalculate the fracture risk to determine whether an individual's risk lies above or below the intervention threshold.
  - high risk – can be considered for treatment without the need for BMD, although BMD measurement may sometimes be appropriate, particularly in younger postmenopausal women.

Technologies SIGN adopted the following position on imaging techniques in 2003 and, in the more recent review, had not identified any further significant evidence leading to any changes to the recommendations:[12]

1 Overall DEXA scanning remains the current standard technique for the diagnosis of osteoporosis due to its ability to measure BMD at a variety of sites.
2 There is insufficient evidence to support the use of any of the other techniques for population screening, or for pre-screening for DEXA.
3 Conventional radiographs should not be used for the diagnosis or exclusion of osteoporosis.

Making recommendations

- From the available data it was estimated that the current DEXA provision should be at least 5000 scans per annum for the whole of Cumbria. However, considering future trends and other evidence it seemed likely that the ideal requirements should be nearer to 9000 scans per annum.[13,14]
- A complete DEXA investigation, including patient preparation, image acquisitions, analysis, printouts and report generation, is typically performed in 20 to 25 minutes, making each DEXA system capable of a throughput of approximately 4000 patients per year.[12] However, the current use of both of the two local scanners was less than this and, in the first instance, it was recommended that the option of increasing productivity be explored.
- However, taking into account geographical factors and the distribution of population density, an additional DEXA scanner may still be required if all communities are to be given equal access. It was therefore also recommended that consideration be given to purchasing a single mobile DEXA scanner for use in a variety of community settings (e.g. community hospitals and large general practices).
- To ensure the appropriate and efficient use of the increased DEXA provision by general practitioners it was recommended that a working group be formed to review and revise the current local guidance (possibly including appropriateness ratings – see next section) and referral forms in relation to the available evidence and guidelines. Furthermore, it was proposed that subsequent DEXA requests by general practitioners be carefully audited against the suggested ratings of 'appropriateness'.

RATING APPROPRIATENESS

The Rand Corporation has a longstanding interest in appropriateness and, in relation to general practitioner-initiated testing, the following definition has been derived from their work: *"for an average group of patients presenting to an average general practitioner clinically appropriate testing means that the expected health benefit(s) exceed the expected negative consequences by a sufficiently wide margin that the test is worth doing".*[15] Moreover, in conjunction with the University of California the Corporation has developed an explicit method to generate appropriateness ratings. The approach entails combining the best scientific evidence with the collective judgement of a group of experts in relation to a list of clinical scenarios.[16] For diagnostic testing this presents an opportunity to produce a series of ratings, on a scale of 1–9, regarding the appropriateness of performing a particular test in relation to patient-specific symptoms, characteristics, medical history and previous investigations.[17]

Currently UK general practitioners are acquiring increased direct access to B-type Natriuretic Peptide (BNP) and echocardiography (Echo) testing with the aim of improving the accuracy of the diagnosis of heart failure. This is partially driven by worries about the overdiagnosis of heart failure by general practitioners who rely simply on the routine clinical assessment (e.g.[18,19]) in circumstances where it might be more appropriate to also arrange a BNP test or echocardiography. For example, many patients with peripheral oedema might, in the absence of diagnostic testing, be labelled as having heart failure when the oedema has another, unrelated aetiology.[20] A further problem that has been highlighted by general practitioners is the difficulty in distinguishing respiratory from cardiac causes of dyspnoea; symptoms of heart failure are often attributed to chronic obstructive pulmonary disease (COPD) and treated incorrectly.[21] However, some have expressed concerns that enhanced access to diagnostic devices might simply lead to more indiscriminate use of BNP with a consequent rise in false positives.[22] As one of the symptoms of heart failure is 'fatigue' it is also quite possible to imagine that the current (and growing) battery of tests ordered by many general practitioners for those who are 'tired all the time' might be extended to include such items as C-reactive protein and BNP (*see* Chapter 9).

Although the Rand Approach has been applied successfully in a number of specialist areas of diagnostic testing (e.g.[23]) no attempt has ever been made to use the method in assessing the appropriateness of diagnostic testing requests by generalists. Therefore, working with a number of colleagues, I sought to develop appropriateness ratings for general practitioners using the Rand Approach in relation to BNP and echocardiography diagnostic testing for possible heart failure.

We first reviewed the literature and generated of a list of 540 clinical scenarios covering the major symptom-initiated presentations within general practice for patients with possible heart failure (but *not* already known to have heart failure). Each scenario was then independently linked to one of three potential decisions that a general practitioner might make:

- **no further investigations (Nil)** – to undertake neither an echocardiogram nor a BNP test
- **echocardiogram (Echo)** – to directly refer for an echocardiogram without undertaking a BNP test
- **BNP triage (BNP)** – to first undertake a BNP test in order to 'rule out' those individuals at low likelihood of heart failure. The remaining patients would subsequently go on to have an echocardiogram.

In addition we identified two recently published systematic reviews covering the relevant evidence, which I obtained and summarised.[7,24]

The 540 scenarios were then ranked, on two occasions, by a panel of general practitioners based on a nine-point scale with 1 indicating 'extremely inappropriate next step' and 9 indicating 'extremely appropriate next step'. In order to combine expertise with external legitimacy, the panel consisted of ten general practitioners, five of whom were GPs with a special interest in cardiology. Furthermore, the panel members were asked to base their ratings on the research evidence in combination with their own clinical experience as general practitioners.[25]

The ratings were then used to generate appropriateness matrices for single symptoms and combinations of symptoms (see below). These illustrate where nothing (nil), BNP testing or Echo were rated the most appropriate (or equally appropriate) next steps.

Finally, as discussed in the previous chapter, there is great potential to apply this approach to other areas of testing uncertainty such as the use of imaging in patients presenting with subjective symptoms of possible oncological significance.

Appropriateness Matrices

Single symptoms:

Cough:

Risk	Exam	ECG	Next steps
			nil
			nil
			BNP
			BNP
			BNP/echo
			echo/BNP

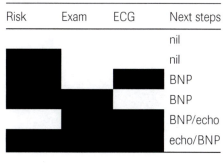

Ankle swelling:

Risk	Exam	ECG	Next steps
			nil
			BNP
			BNP
			BNP
			BNP
			BNP
			BNP/echo*

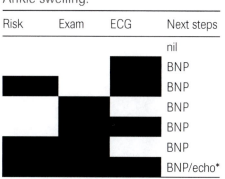

Dyspnoea:

Risk	Exam	ECG	Next steps
			BNP
			BNP
			BNP
			BNP
			BNP/echo
			BNP/echo*
			echo/BNP

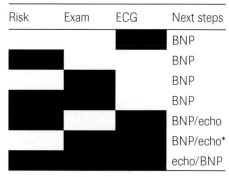

Fatigue:

Risk	Exam	ECG	Next steps
			Nil
			BNP
			BNP
			BNP/echo*
			echo/BNP

Symptom combinations:

Cough and Ankle Swelling:

Risk	Exam	ECG	Next steps
			nil
			BNP
			BNP
			BNP
			BNP/echo
			BNP/echo*
			echo/BNP

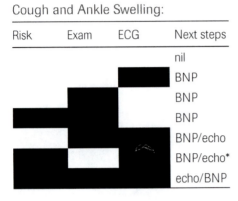

Ankle swelling and Dyspnoea:

Risk	Exam	ECG	Next steps
			BNP
			BNP
			BNP
			BNP/echo
			BNP/echo*
			BNP/echo
			echo/BNP

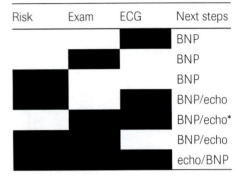

Cough and Dyspnoea:

Risk	Exam	ECG	Next steps
			nil
			BNP
			BNP
			BNP
			BNP/echo*
			BNP/echo*
			echo/BNP

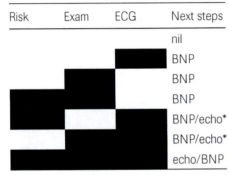

Ankle swelling and fatigue:

Risk	Exam	ECG	Next steps
			nil
			BNP
			BNP
			BNP
			BNP/echo
			echo/BNP

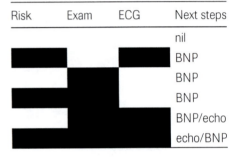

Cough and Fatigue:

Risk	Exam	ECG	Next steps
			nil
			BNP
			BNP/echo*
			echo/BNP

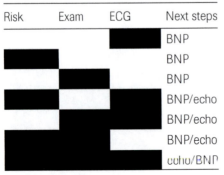

Cough, Ankle swelling and Dyspnoea:

Risk	Exam	ECG	Next steps
			BNP
			BNP
			BNP
			BNP
			BNP/echo
			BNP/echo
			BNP/echo
			echo/BNP

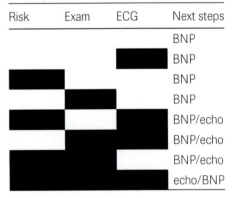

Fatigue and Dyspnoea:

Risk	Exam	ECG	Next steps
			BNP
			BNP
			BNP
			BNP/echo
			BNP/echo
			BNP/echo
			echo/BNP

Cough, Ankle swelling and Fatigue:

Risk	Exam	ECG	Next steps
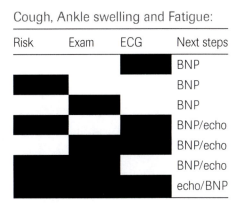

BNP
BNP
BNP
BNP/echo
BNP/echo
BNP/echo
echo/BNP

Fatigue, Ankle swelling and Dyspnoea:

Risk	Exam	ECG	Next steps
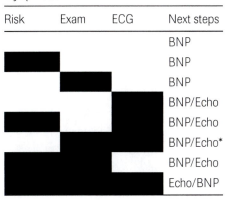

BNP
BNP
BNP
BNP/Echo
BNP/Echo
BNP/Echo*
BNP/Echo
Echo/BNP

Cough, Fatigue and Dyspnoea:

Risk	Exam	ECG	Next steps
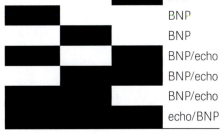

BNP
BNP
BNP
BNP/echo
BNP/echo
BNP/echo
echo/BNP

Cough, Fatigue, Ankle swelling and Dyspnoea:

Risk	Exam	ECG	Next steps
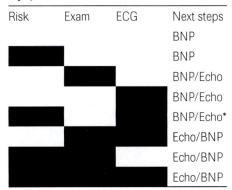

BNP
BNP
BNP/Echo
BNP/Echo
BNP/Echo*
Echo/BNP
Echo/BNP
Echo/BNP

KEY

Risk = Cardiovascular risk (low/intermediate vs high)

Exam = Cardiovascular/chest examination (normal vs abnormal)

ECG = ECG (normal vs abnormal/none)

- ■ *Abnormal finding or high cardiovascular risk*
- □ *Normal finding or low/intermediate cardiovascular risk*
- • **Echocardiogram (Echo)** – to directly refer for an echocardiogram without undertaking a BNP test.
- • **BNP triage (BNP)** – to first undertake a BNP/NT-proBNP test in order to 'rule out' those individuals at low likelihood of heart failure.

In the matrices, the following sequence applies:

BNP/Echo = BNP is the most appropriate next step

Echo/BNP = Echo is the most appropriate next step

BNP/Echo* = BNP and echo are seen as equally appropriate next steps

GENERAL REFERENCES

- Knottnerus JA, Buntinx F. *The Evidence Base of Clinical Diagnosis.* Oxford: Wiley-Blackwell, 2009.

TEXT REFERENCES

1. Summerton AM, Summerton N. The use of desk-top cholesterol analysers in general practice. *Public Health* 1995; **109**: 363–7.
2. Mant J, Fitzmaurice DA, Hobbs FDR, *et al.* Accuracy of diagnosing atrial fibrillation on electrocardiogram by primary care practitioners and interpretative diagnostic software: analysis of data from screening for atrial fibrillation in the elderly (SAFE) trial. *BMJ* 2007; **335**: 380–5.
3. Strong M, South G, Carlisle R. The UK Quality and Outcomes Framework pay-for-performance scheme and spirometry: rewarding quality or just quantity? A cross-sectional study in Rotherham, UK. *BMC Health Services Research* 2009; **9**: 108–15.
4. National Imaging Board. *Ultrasound Clinical Governance.* London: DH, 2008.
5. Auditor General for Scotland. *Review of NHS Diagnostic Services.* Edinburgh: Audit Scotland, 2008.
6. Glasziou PP, Irwig L, Heritier S, *et al.* Monitoring cholesterol levels: measurement error or true change? *Ann Intern Med* 2008; **148**: 656–61.
7. Mant J, Doust J, Roalfe A, *et al.* Systematic review and individual patient data meta-analysis of diagnosis for heart failure, with modelling of implications of different diagnostic strategies in primary care. *Health Technology Assessment* 2009; **13**: 32.
8. Widjaja E, Manuel D, Hodgson TJ, *et al.* Imaging findings and referral outcomes of rapid assessment stroke clinics. *Clinical Radiology* 2005; **60**: 1076–82.
9. www.shef.ac.uk/FRAX/tool.jsp?locationValue=1
10. Lord SJ, Irwig L, Simes RJ. When is measuring sensitivity and specificity sufficient to evaluate a diagnostic test, and when do we need randomized trials? *Ann Intern Med* 2006; **144**: 850–5.
11. Sambrook P, Cooper C. Osteoporosis: trends in epidemiology, pathogenesis and treatment. *Lancet* 2006; **367**: 2010–18.
12. Scottish Intercollegiate Guidelines Network. *Management of osteoporosis. A National Clinical Guideline.* Edinburgh: SIGN, 2003 (reviewed 2007).
13. Rowe RE, Cooper CC. Osteoporosis services in secondary care: a UK survey. *J Roy Soc Med* 2000; **93**: 22–4.
14. Thomas E, Richardson JC, Irvine A, *et al.* Osteoporosis: what are the implications of scanning 'high risk' women in primary care? *Family Practice* 2003; **20**: 289–93.
15. Brook RH. Appropriateness: the next frontier. *BMJ* 1994; **308**: 218–19.
16. Hicks NR. Some observations on attempts to measure appropriateness of care. *BMJ* 1994; **309**: 730–3.
17. Fitch K, Bernstein SJ, Aguilar MD, *et al. The RAND/UCLA Appropriateness Method User's Manual.* The Rand Corporation: Santa Monica, CA; 2001 www.rand.org/pubs/monograph_reports/MR1269/index.html
18. Remes J, Miettinen H, Reunanen A, Pyorala K. Validity of clinical diagnosis of heart failure in primary healthcare. *European Heart Journal* 1991; **12**: 315–21.
19. Wheeldon NM, MacDonald TM, Flucker CJ, *et al.* Echocardiography in chronic heart failure in the community. *Quarterly Journal of Medicine* 1993; **86**: 17–23.

20. Blankfield RP, Finkelhor RS, Alexander JJ, *et al*. Etiology and diagnosis of bilateral leg edema in primary care. *Am J Med* 1998; **105**: 192–7.

21. Mogelvang R, Goetze JP, Schnohr P, *et al*. Discriminating between cardiac and pulmonary dysfunction in the general population with dyspnoea by plasma pro-B-type natriuretic peptide. *J Am Coll Cardiol* 2007; **50**: 1694–701.

22. Heart Improvement Programme. *Brain-type Natriuretic Peptide (BNP)*. An Information Resource for Cardiac Networks. NHS Improvement, 2008.

23. ACCF Appropriateness Criteria Working Group. ACCF/ASNC Appropriateness Criteria for Single-Photon Emission Computed Tomography Myocardial Perfusion Imaging (SPECT MPI). *J Am Coll Cardiol* 2005; **46**: 1587–605.

24. Madhok V, Falk G, Rogers A, *et al*. The accuracy of symptoms, signs and diagnostic tests in the diagnosis of left ventricular dysfunction in primary care: A diagnostic accuracy systematic review. *BMC Family Practice* 2008; **6**: 56.

25. Campbell SM, Fuat A, Summerton N, *et al*. Diagnostic triage and the role of natriuretic peptide and echocardiography for suspected heart failure: an appropriateness ratings evaluation by UK general practitioners. *Brit J Gen Pract* (in press).

CHAPTER 11

Conclusion

As has been discussed throughout this book, primary care diagnostics concerns the interpretation and the rational application of information obtained directly from the patient. It is about re-emphasising the importance of the patient's input into the diagnostic process and performing investigations only after careful consideration has been given to the costs and the benefits as viewed from the patient's perspective. Furthermore, the ultimate value of any diagnostic processing must be judged in relation to patient-oriented and health service outcomes.

Primary care diagnostics should also be based on the best available scientific evidence applicable to the primary care context. However, this does not mean that such evidence is the only issue that matters. Clinical experience and clinical wisdom are also critical components of the primary care approach. Sometimes it is simply a matter of not losing our nerve in a situation of uncertainty or rushing to undertake inappropriate investigations.

Thus I propose that eight fundamental features constitute primary care diagnostics:

1 maintaining a broad and patient-centred approach
2 being alert to the importance of context and its impact on the validity and the reliability of all clinical information
3 using information obtained from the medical history and the clinical examination wisely
4 harnessing the diagnostic processing pathway both for clinical care and for commissioning
5 focusing on patient-oriented and health service outcomes
6 appreciating the unique nature of primary care decision making in relation to, for example, precision and uncertainty
7 adopting distinct diagnostic strategies such as the 'test of time'
8 ensuring the appropriate and efficient use of investigations combined with clarity about the purpose of any test

When I work my way through a busy surgery, I attempt to keep the issues discussed in this book foremost in my mind. However, although I believe that I have managed to enhance the quality and the quantity of the input I receive from patients, rarely is there enough time to explicitly apply Bayes' Theorem or to discuss risks and decision-making thresholds with patients. Research has also demonstrated that the question, "Did the doctor give you chance to say what was really on your mind?" was more likely to be answered in the affirmative in the context of longer consultations. Thus, for me, primary care diagnostics also raises two fundamental questions about the way we use our limited healthcare resources:

1 Should commissioners of healthcare consider funding more primary care clinical time as an alternative to yet more new diagnostic technologies?
2 Should primary care physicians focus more on diagnostics, and some of their other tasks be re-assigned to other members of the primary healthcare team?

Glossary

Bayes' Theorem (odds ratio form)
A theorem that permits the calculation of the posterior odds of a disease by knowing the prior odds of the disease and the likelihood ratio of the clinical indicant being used.

$$\text{posterior odds} = \text{prior odds} \times \text{likelihood ratio}$$

Clinical indicant
Items or combinations of items of clinical information indicating the likely presence or absence of a condition.

Clinical information
Symptoms, features in the medical history, patient characteristics (e.g. age, sex) and information derived from the clinical examination or as a result of investigations (tests).

Discriminant value
An assessment of the capacity of a clinical indicant to distinguish between two or more outcomes. Measures of a clinical indicant's discriminant value include predictive value, sensitivity, specificity and likelihood ratio.

Likelihood ratio
The likelihood that a given result in relation to the clinical information would be expected in a patient with the disease compared to the likelihood that the same result would be expected in a patient without the disease. Likelihood ratios indicate how many times more (or less) likely a result is in a patient with the disease compared to a patient free of disease.

likelihood ratio

$$= \frac{\text{proportion of patients } \textit{with} \text{ disease and } \textit{with} \text{ clinical finding}}{\text{proportion of patients } \textit{without} \text{ disease and } \textit{with} \text{ clinical finding}}$$

positive likelihood ratio

$$= \frac{\text{proportion of patients } \textit{with} \text{ disease and } \textit{with} \text{ positive clinical finding}}{\text{proportion of patients } \textit{without} \text{ disease and } \textit{with} \text{ positive clinical finding}}$$

negative likelihood ratio

$$= \frac{\text{proportion of patients } \textit{with} \text{ disease and } \textit{with} \text{ negative clinical finding}}{\text{proportion of patients } \textit{without} \text{ disease and } \textit{with} \text{ negative clinical finding}}$$

Odds
The ratio of the likelihood of the event occurring over the likelihood of the event not occurring.

$$\text{odds} = \frac{\text{probability}}{1\text{-probability}}$$

Positive predictive value
The probability that the disease is present if the clinical indicant is positive [present]. (The negative predictive value is the probability that the disease is absent if the clinical indicant is negative, [absent]).

Posterior odds
The odds of an event conditional upon another event having occurred.

Prior odds
The odds of an event before acquiring additional information.

Probability
A number that expresses an opinion about the likelihood of an event.

$$\text{probability} = \frac{\text{odds}}{1 + \text{odds}}$$

Receiver operator characteristic (ROC) curve
A graphic representation of the relationship between the true-positive rate of a clinical indicant and the false-positive rate of the same clinical indicant as the criterion (cut-off point) of a positive result is changed.

Reference standard
The procedure that is used to define the true state of the patient.

Reliability
The extent to which repeated measurements of a stable phenomenon produce similar results (also 'reproducibility').

Screening
The presumptive identification of unrecognised disease or defects by the application of tests, examinations, or other procedures that can be applied rapidly.

Sensitivity

The probability of a positive result in relation to the clinical information if the disease is present (the 'true-positive' rate).

Specificity

The probability of a negative result in relation to the clinical information if the disease is absent (the 'true-negative' rate).

Index